ON CALL
by
Sandra Hoynacki

CHAPTER ONE

I walked into the diner and sat down in the corner booth. The sun hid behind the clouds as if it wanted no part of this meeting or the ridiculous bet that brought me here. The waitress came over with a glass of water and took my order. I felt sure she would rather be anywhere but here. Similar feelings gnawed within me. A foolish thought crossed my mind: *I should look at myself in the mirror to see if I am presentable. Maybe add a little lipstick or powder. Stop being ridiculous*, I mumbled to myself. *Who cares what I look like at a time like this?* I don't even know why I bothered to show up. In any minute, they would walk in the door—total strangers with the power to change my world forever. Kathy had been vague about the meeting. She was my best friend, but she was always complaining of boredom. Sometimes, I wanted to strangle her.

The waitress placed apple pie and coffee in front of me. Between the heat of the day and the pending meeting, the thought of eating made me nauseous. The door opened and in walked two normal-looking individuals. One was dressed in a business suit while the other wore a sport jacket and khakis. Why did Kathy suggest this in fun when a full-blown nightmare danced on the proverbial stage?

They glanced around casually before strolling toward me. Chills of fear clutched every part of me. I couldn't explain the evil that I felt overshadowing me.

They nodded in unison as they slid into the booth opposite me. Maybe they thought they were being inconspicuous, but I think the expression on my face must've spoken volumes about the irregularity of our meeting. Avoiding all niceties, they cut straight to the interrogation.

"Have you figured out the situation yet?" the sharp-dressed male asked. His voice was emotionless and his eyes were darker than his demeanor.

"Yes, I believe I have." I replied, hoping to sound like I knew what they were referring to. "Let's get to the facts. I want this over quickly."
I took a sip of my coffee and sat back, trying to play it cool. Mr. Dark Eyes wasn't fazed by me.

"It would benefit you, Miss, to be aware of all of our expectations since there are others whose lives may depend on it. Just to be sure that we are on the same page, give me an idea of why you think this meeting is taking place, or do you even have a clue?"

Geez, this guy means business. Looks like Mr. Dark Eyes was chosen to do all the talking. All the while his partner stared down at my pie. *Should I offer to call over the waitress so he could order himself some food? No! Just answer him and get this meeting over!*

"As I said before, I understand the situation. I believe you are here offering me extra money so that I will be prepared to go at a moment's notice or whenever staff doctors deem it necessary to call me in."

"Okay, good. Please refrain from speaking about this to anyone." He paused. "It's to your benefit to understand that, Miss."

I restrained the urge to roll my eyes at him. *Why does he keep calling me "Miss" like that? How creepy!* Maybe I was scared to death, but I wasn't about to let them in on that fact.

"As far as I am concerned, Sir, we don't have a contractual agreement. The limitations placed on me are ridiculous. You want to call the shots, write the policies and incorporate any rules that benefit whatever the agenda may be while leaving me in the dark concerning God knows what."

He took a deep breath and I could tell by the darkening of his already black eyes that my comments were not appreciated. His silent partner straightened up in his seat, excitedly waiting for the snake to shoot his venom at me.

"You're here, aren't you, little lady? You have, indeed, concluded by now that this meeting wasn't a Sunday afternoon tête-à-tête with the girls from work. You wouldn't be here if you didn't want the money. The contract is just a formality. You've already made up your mind."

I fidgeted in my seat as the men glared at me. I faced a dangerous situation. These tough guys, in charge of a sordid scheme and displaying the cockiness of the Mafia, had total control. The rules had already been written, and there were no options. I could play their game or go home, but even that wasn't a possibility anymore. I was in too deep and there was no turning back now.

Waves of apprehension swept over me, but I didn't dare flinch. I would not give them the pleasure of seeing me squirm. As I passively stared back at them, fear shook every fiber within me.

"What time does the….uh…the product need to be placed in the container for pick-up?" I asked.

"Someone will call you at the hospital next week, on Wednesday to be precise."

His partner gave him a nod to confirm the day.

"You'll always be paid in cash," he added.

As if any of these kinds of transactions were ever paid with a Visa! I thought to myself sarcastically.

Mr. Dark Eyes motioned to his buddy that it was time to go. He stopped briefly and leaned closer to whisper his final threat.

"And one more thing, Miss, don't *ever* try to contact any of us."

My eyes locked on both faces. I wondered why a couple of well-groomed men in their late thirties decided to settle here. I froze at the thought of what was happening inside the cozy little mom-and-pop town of Morganville, California.

The two men left as leisurely as they had arrived. Inside my gut, a wall of fear gnawed at me. Kathy and I were undoubtedly involved in something sinister. We were going to be on call for these people, and yet, the players behind this game remained anonymous. Numbness took over. *Why did Kathy involve me in this?*

CHAPTER TWO

Daddy and Mama brought me up in a modest town much like Morganville. Sidewalks were rolled up by nine at night. Folks left their doors unlocked. Our picturesque community catered to seniors and weekly gabfests. After I graduated from nursing school, life in the small town became stagnant, and I became restless.

Moving to a new location where I could find a stable job and maybe even find love was the logical way out. I talked with my parents and we agreed on the town where I would relocate, along with the date of my departure.

The move to Morganville proved to be a wise decision. I found a nursing job at the local hospital within a few weeks. I earned a promotion after six months on the job. The administrator respected flexibility and results. He spoke highly of me to staff doctors. Kathy had been charge nurse in previous positions and filled in for me if needed for meetings and such. We had a lot in common, which contributed to our being best friends right from the start. Kathy was a hard-working, intellectually-blessed, and adventurous individual. She kidded me often, saying I was a straight-laced Victorian nurse and a prude.

If only I had listened to my inner "prude" and avoided taking Kathy up on her bet to come to the diner for this meeting. She called to remind me about it last night; otherwise, I might have forgotten. While it was true that Kathy's game playing had the potential to enhance our bank accounts, I was beginning to wonder if it would be worth it. I only decided to follow through with this bet since I thought no harm could come of it. A verbal guarantee of substantial salary increases seemed a bit strange in my book since most business deals didn't occur in this manner. However, neither of us questioned the extra work; after all, the hospital employed us.

As I stirred my cold coffee, I attempted to figure out what had just taken place. In broad daylight, two nameless characters had suddenly appeared and demanded…

The more I stirred, the angrier I became. That anger mixed with anxiety. As the combination rose up inside of me, I responded by throwing the spoon down on the table. The waitress shot a disgusted look at me from her place at the end of the counter. I stood abruptly and allowed the door to slam behind me as I left the diner.

My high heels clicked loudly on the concrete as I stormed toward my car. The sound sent birds scattering in every direction. *Why did I park near a dark alley a block away from civilization?* I asked myself. As I approached my car, I could feel sweat clinging to my skin like a wet coat. I anxiously peered into the back seat, which offered a perfect hiding place for an unsavory character. I had to make a decision: continue into the car or turn back to the diner and face the long walk home. *Walk? In these heels? No way!* I noticed the sun was painting a backdrop of shadows on the pavement. After a quick inspection, I was certain there was no one in the car; so I eased into my vehicle.

I turned the key in the ignition and wondered if the thugs who threatened me knew where I lived. Maybe they were connected to the mysterious events that had plagued my life over the past few months.

My mind drifted in many directions as I pulled into traffic. Kathy mentioned that the extra work was in a surgical unit doing organ retrievals. Suddenly, it occurred to me that the trafficking of human organs had been making headlines. I thought back to an article that I recently read concerning money flow on the black market. *Is this what I just signed up for?* The thought made me ill.

The drive home felt like it took forever. Of course it didn't help that I felt the need to glance in my rear-view mirror every five seconds to make sure I wasn't being followed. Was I overreacting?

With sweaty palms, I unlocked the door in a frenzy. The light from the ringing phone flashed like a generic Morse code. My keys fell to the floor as I ran across the living room in an attempt to grab the receiver, but I was too late. The answering machine had already picked up.

"Jenny, this is Kathy! I must speak with you..... This is an emergency, please pick up!"

I stopped myself from picking up the phone when I heard her message. *How dare she try to act concerned now!* I flung the cabinet door open, hitting the back wall. Glasses tumbled out and crashed against the kitchen floor. Tears streamed down my face. I opened the pantry to get the broom and a mouse scampered across the top of my feet.

Damn Kathy and her "Alice in Wonderland" personality. There wasn't a suspicious bone in her body. I couldn't say the same about mine.

A Valium would settle my nerves. I needed to place things in the proper perspective. If I could at least make sense of what transpired at the diner, maybe my fears would lessen.

It was getting dark. My stomach didn't normally churn like this. I mixed a Scotch and water. The swirling of the ice against the side of the glass was soothing. The shrill ringing of the phone brought me to reality once again.

"Hello, Jenny?" asked the male voice.

"Yes, who is calling?" I responded trying not to sound frazzled. I was expecting it to be Kathy again and I was ready to unleash my wrath on her.

"Jenny, this is Dr. Kenalog at the Morganville Hospital."

"Oh, Dr. Kenalog, you've never called me at home before. I didn't recognize your voice, sir." I took a breath.

"Jenny, I need you to be at the hospital in the morning at six o'clock sharp. We have an accident case and need to get started on it immediately." "Yes, sir, Doctor. I'll be there." I paused, but he didn't respond. "Uh, goodbye, sir."

The dial tone was the next sound that I heard. *How did he know to call me? Why did he hang up so abruptly? Oh no, could it be that he...?*

The receiver fell from my hand and hit the floor with a thud. I wondered how this man could do this. He was a doctor who took the Hippocratic Oath to save lives and ... and... but, wait a minute. I was jumping to conclusions. No one had done a thing yet. *Had they?* The phone was beeping loudly as it lay on the floor. Maybe leaving it off the hook for the remainder of the night would help to alleviate my fears. I was headed to the bedroom when it hit me: The phone was not the problem. That had nothing to do with any of this. Trembling, I put the receiver on the hook and sat down on the couch.

Dr. Kenalog was the Director of the Organ Retrieval Program and Director of the Medical Examiner's Office. Come to think of it, he seemed to be involved in all of the cases where the accident victims died from their injuries. My nerves began to tighten like a cord. I felt as if I were at my breaking point. My imagination was working overtime. I had no proof of anything.

I made up my mind to call Kathy, only to reach her voice mail. There wasn't a need to leave a message. What would I say to her anyway?

The Valium and Scotch were working on me in an unusual way. My stomach was empty. The last time I could remember eating was at the diner, and I didn't finish the pie.

The room started spinning as a hot, smothering sensation came over me. The couch was spinning out of reach. I was feeling weak, and there was nothing to sit on. I made it to the bedroom door and somehow staggered onto my bed. Sleep was all that mattered, not thinking. I was too tired to think…

I awoke with a throbbing headache and a nauseated stomach. I wasn't sure of the time or how long I was asleep. *Why do I still have on the same clothes that I wore yesterday? Ah, yes,* I remembered. Anger began to rise inside of me. I made a decision that might cause my demise. The ringing phone startled me.

"Hello, is this Jenny?" asked the caller.

"Yes, who ... who is this?" I asked hesitantly.

"This is Code Blue Search," responded the monotone voice.

"What?" I stammered. "What did you say?"

"You heard me. Code Blue Search. Now just listen. We had scheduled a meeting for next week but those plans have changed. You will be doing a case this morning at six. You will take the necessary steps to compensate for this change of plans. The arrangements for pickup will take place within two hours of your call to a number I'm going to give you. When you call the number, you will be given instructions for the next move. Do you understand?"

I stood still with my mouth gaping. *What have I gotten myself into?*

"Yes, I....I...who....the..." I couldn't even put my thoughts together to make a complete sentence.

"The number is 206-2348."

I leaped over to my bedside table to grab a pen. Suddenly the phone died. The silence was deafening.

Code Blue was the term used by the medical team in cases where the possibility of a patient dying was present. I wondered what the "Search" part meant. *What were they looking for... what or... oh, my God, where was I headed?*

It was a good thing that the bed was behind me. The heaving started from deep down in my stomach and made its way to my throat. Waves of sickness came over me. The bathroom was close. My guts felt like they were exploding.

CHAPTER THREE

Before long, it was time to get cleaned up and ready for work. I needed to be there at six. The room was still spinning. I wasn't sure that I could physically do what I had to do. A shower would make me feel better. *I have to do this...I don't have a choice.* I staggered into the bathroom and ran the water for a few seconds. After a long day at the hospital, a long, relaxing shower or bubble bath was the one luxury that I had always afforded myself, but this wasn't the time for my usual lengthy aquatic therapy.

The water felt good streaming down my face and body. It would clean the stench that had invaded me without invitation. The shower perked me up. It gave me the strength I needed to get dressed. I pulled on my freshly-starched uniform combined with stockings and polished shoes. I was actually starting to feel like a human being again.

Thankfully, I recently had my hair cut short, so it didn't take me as long to get ready in the morning. Still, I was very particular about styling it so that it stayed just right throughout the day. It was important to me to look my best, especially at a time like this. I fixed my nursing hat carefully atop my dark auburn hair. Though other nurses complained about wearing it, I was more than happy for my uniform to be complete. And besides, I worked hard to earn this hat; so I would wear it regardless of the rules. Of course, this was one of Kathy's favorite picking points.

She just loved to tease me about my obsession with my hair (and my hat).

Food was the last thing on my mind. It wouldn't stay in my stomach for long anyway. Maybe just coffee would be enough to get me started. One final check in the mirror and I was ready to go. *Deep breaths,* I reminded myself. I dug the keys out of my purse and headed toward the door.

The street was deserted, but I felt the strangest urge to look around before I stepped outside. Paranoia was a big part of my nature, like breathing. I wasn't one to take risks. This whole scenario was completely out of character for me. *What have I gotten myself into?* I questioned myself for the thousandth time.

I climbed into my car, wondering if anyone was watching me. It was still dark outside, and fear was riding on my shoulders. I made sure the doors were locked. It was only a few miles to the hospital.

Who would know if something happened to me? Would Kathy know to look for me if...if....? What would Mom and Dad do if I got hurt? I was in a daze.

Suddenly there were red and blue lights blinking behind me. A police car was coming up on my bumper. I pulled over to the side of the road hoping he would pass me, but of course, I wasn't having that kind of good fortune these days. *Darn.*

I lowered my window as the officer approached my vehicle.

"Ma'am, Do you know why I pulled you over?" He asked as though he'd rehearsed the line in his sleep.

"Uh, no sir. I don't believe I was speeding or anything." *Was I?* I really wasn't sure about anything at this point.

"Actually, you *were* speeding *and* you ran the four-way stop back there." He seemed angered and quite certain about his accusations. He waited somewhat patiently for my pitiful defense.

"Sir, I didn't... I mean I saw...I....I…"

It was obvious that I was having problems making any sense. He could tell that I was upset or maybe he suspected I was on drugs. The tears that forced their way into my eyes made them a bit glassy.

"Are you okay?" His stance softened a bit.

"Yes sir, I am. I had my mind on something else." *I think I'm involved in the trafficking of human organs. But really, it's no big deal.* "I'm sorry. I know you've got to give me a ticket, but I need to hurry and get to work. I'll be more careful sir, I promise."

I couldn't help but hope that in seeing a distressed nurse with her hat on, he might be infused with a tinge of compassion. He scratched his head and shifted his weight back and forth, as if he was balancing the scales of justice. He scribbled something onto his notepad, and then he handed me a warning ticket. *Whew!* I thanked him and promised once more that it wouldn't happen again. The officer walked back to his car and seemed satisfied that he did his good deed for the day by letting me go. I wholeheartedly agreed. I was definitely in need of a break.

For the remainder of the short ride, I felt like I was in some sort of a vacuum. The parking lot at the hospital looked dismal and deserted. Fog surrounded the building like a shroud. *Where's the guard? Why are all the lights out in the parking lot?* I felt anxious and was regretting my decision to skip breakfast.

The elevator took forever to reach the sixth floor. The door opened, and as I stepped out, I saw the orderly from the morgue pushing a gurney into operating room number six. This had to be the donor on the doctor's list.

Maybe another cup of coffee would help. I walked to the nurses' lounge. I usually limit myself to two cups of coffee; more than that and I get the jitters. But that didn't matter to me at the moment. Sleep is a necessity when working in an operating room. Though I passed out last night, I wouldn't exactly call that a restful night's sleep. I was struggling to keep my eyes open.

Suddenly a voice startled me. I jumped, spun around, and the man's eyes met mine.

I was face to face with the voice from last night's phone call.

"Good morning, Jenny, how are you?" he asked nonchalantly.

"I'm fine, Dr. Kenalog, and you, sir?" I replied trying to duplicate his coolness.

"I'm ready to go. Get scrubbed and meet me in O.R. number six," he answered.

He was gone before I had a chance to ask him any further questions.

The back table in the operating room was set for the procedure. All of the instruments had been placed in the correct order. Several team members were there, fully gowned, scrubbed and ready for their part, including Dr. Kenalog.

Suddenly I couldn't move my feet; they felt as if they were frozen in place. Kathy stood near the table staring at me over her mask. Her marble eyes spoke volumes to me. She looked as though the devil himself was standing behind her. I managed to take my position beside her and waited for the doctor to begin. We would be harvesting the bones and lymph nodes. That was the extent of what Kathy and I knew.

The patient, a middle-aged man, was listed only as an accident victim. He didn't appear to be physically injured, which left even more questions looming. The doctor took his position at the table. He asked for the scalpel. The removal of the organs began. The tissue was excised and placed on the back table. The standard procedure was to place the tissue in preservatives before transport.

No one was talking. When the body was turned, I noted that there were no noticeable scratches or bruises. I turned to look at Kathy as the doctor motioned to his colleague, whom I didn't know or recognize as a doctor on our staff. Everything that was happening was illegal. The name of the deceased had been changed. Dr. Kenalog stated that our team would be known as "The Code Blue Search Group," and we were under explicit orders not to speak of anything that happened in the operating room.

We were sinking deeper into the muck of dishonesty and couldn't do one thing about it. I wondered what Kathy thought of her little bet now. No amount of money would make up for the things that we would become involved in from this day forth.

We finished the accident case. Someone else picked up the containers I was responsible for retrieving. A physician came into the operating room and took my place. Kathy and I were asked to leave. The new face at the back table and a few select staff were the only ones allowed to assist with the closing.

I left the operating area and headed to the nurses' lounge. Getting out of there was the only thing on my mind. Kathy stared at me as if she was in a trance.

I sensed she wanted to talk, but my anger was building towards Kathy as well as myself. Previous to this day, I had always made sound decisions.

I stormed past Kathy in the hallway in front of the operating room. Just beyond the elevator door, a shadow loomed overhead on the far side of the wall. I stopped walking. Fear prevented me from taking another step. I turned and ran back in the direction of the operating rooms.

I busted through the doors of the room where the procedure had been performed. I found Kathy talking to Dr. Kenalog. *Oh no!* They swiftly turned to face me. My momentum kept me moving forward. *I need to get out of here!* My thoughts were shouting inside my head. When I turned, Kathy reached out to me. I was out of breath and couldn't feel my legs. The room started spinning, and blackness quietly took over.

CHAPTER FOUR

My eyes were closed and I could feel the cold, hard floor underneath me. I heard a distant voice through the fogginess. Maybe this was all a bad dream.

"Jenny, Jenny, wake up, talk to me." Kathy's voice echoed in my head.

The bottle of scents was pungent. I pushed it out of my face and tried to sit up.

"Where am I?" My eyes were still trying to focus on the face in front of me.

"You are in the recovery room. You fainted in the hallway just outside the O.R. Don't you remember?" Kathy asked.

She felt my forehead and brushed my hair away from my face. *God only knows what I must look like right now! I've never fainted in all my life.*

"No, I was going to the elevator, and there was a … never mind. Help me get up. I have to get out of here!" I was adamant.

"Wait, I need to talk to you, Jenny. Can we go for coffee or something?"

"No, we can't," I responded. Despite my answer, Kathy helped me to stand up. I tried to fix my hair and straighten out my uniform. "I'm too angry to discuss this with you."

"But that is why we need…" Kathy looked at me pathetically through her long eyelashes.

I could never tell if I was being manipulated by her or if she was just oblivious to her charms. Regardless, this time I was determined to stand my ground and not let her get away with it. I held up my hand to stop her mid-sentence.

"Good-bye, Kathy."

I stormed out of the operating room and headed to the main elevator that led to the busier part of the hospital. It was usually bustling with people and I felt it would be safe.

In the elevator, a couple of nurses were discussing their boyfriends. A few doctors got on at the next floor. I stepped to the back of the elevator and stood silently. The elevator filled up quickly. I was the only occupant who wasn't busy chatting about unimportant things. I wondered what they would think if they knew what was going on in this well-known hospital.

I saw nothing unusual when I stepped into the lobby. No one was watching me as far as I could tell. A wave of relief came over me as I headed to the parking lot. It was early afternoon and I had time to do my grocery shopping. I got in the car, put the keys in the ignition, and buckled my seat belt. The radio came on when I started the car. The news shot out at me like a bolt of lightning.

"It has just been learned that there was an attempted prison break at midmorning today. The National Guard had to be called in to halt the riots. We also have reports that several prisoners were injured or killed.

Please stay tuned for further information on the afternoon news."

I suddenly felt sick. There hadn't been a prison break in years. I talked to Kathy about that right after we became friends. This was a big concern of mine because I lived within a few miles of the prison. I had found my apartment after a short search. I immediately fell in love with it. It was located across the street from a beautiful park. I knew the prison was there, but Kathy assured me that there were never any incidents.

My mind was churning as I drove to the grocery store. My head felt as if it would burst. I parked the car and headed towards the store. When my cell phone rang, I reached into my purse and turned it off. It was Kathy. I decided not to answer it. I wasn't going to talk to her. She could leave a message.

I rushed into the store. It seemed like an eternity since all of this began. I wondered about the problem at the prison. I grabbed a few items and headed to the check-out line. While waiting there, I noticed the girl who'd worked the back table at the hospital standing across the aisle talking to the produce clerk. I watched her for a moment and decided to look down and ignore her. I was confused, angry, and, above all, scared. Suddenly, I heard a voice call my name. It was her.

"Hi, you're Jenny, right?" the bubbly young nurse asked as she got in line behind me.

"Yes, uh-huh, I am Jenny. I don't believe I caught your name." I pretended I hadn't noticed her.

"Chloe Evans. I'm new in town. I don't know anyone yet. I did meet your friend Kathy a couple of days ago." She smiled at the young man at the register who was scanning my items.

You mean my ex-friend? "Uh, yes, Kathy and I are very good friends. I've only been at the hospital about a year. Where are you from, Chloe?" *I wonder whose side she's on—theirs or ours.*

"New York. My parents run a couple of businesses there. They asked me to come here and help Dr. Kenalog; so here I am." Chloe posed like a cheerleader prepped for the big game.

Dr. Kenalog, huh? I guess that answers that— she's on their side.

"What kind of businesses do your parents own in New York?" I acted genuinely interested while the register beeped with my total.

"Oh, they have the largest funeral home in New York, and they also manage the biomedical lab and the crematorium on the outskirts of the city."

I gulped as I swiped my card to pay. *Did she say funeral home? Deep breaths,* I reminded myself.

"What do your parents do?" she asked.

Chloe barely looked up as she picked through the gum selection. I typed in my pin number and choked out a response.

"Uh, my dad is a retired naval officer and Mom is a C.P.A. at a small business in Canyonville."

She nodded but I doubt that she was paying attention. The cashier held out my receipt.

"I need to be going now, Chloe. I'll see you again at the hospital, I'm sure. Take care, okay?" I picked up my bags and didn't look back.

"Okay, nice to meet you Jenny," she called out.

I couldn't get to my car fast enough. I was more afraid than ever before. I felt sure I was going to be killed at any moment, even though it was broad daylight. The prison breaks, the new girl whose parents sent her here from New York to harvest organs... What was going on in this wholesome town? Would Hell open up and swallow us into our own nightmare—a nightmare that we were involved in creating?

CHAPTER FIVE

I enjoyed my Saturday mornings' routine: reading the paper in bed with my coffee and smelling fresh-baked donuts from the bakery on the corner. It was my personal leisure time. I got out of bed and cracked open the window. Joggers were in the park across the street. The city workers just mowed the luscious green grass, and I could smell its sweet fragrance from the spot where I stood.

I prepared the coffee pot the night before, so all I needed to do was push the button to start the brewing. I walked to the front door and picked up the paper. When the coffee was ready, I poured a cupful and got back into bed.

The prison events of the previous day made the front page. Three deaths were linked to the attempted jail break. I knew what that meant: prisoners, if qualified, could donate organs for transplants.

After a hot shower, I felt better. I decided this was the perfect day to take a bike ride in the park. Just as I stepped out of the bathroom, the phone rang. I quickly wrapped my wet hair up in a towel and answered it.

"Hello," I said into the receiver.

"Jenny, this is Kathy, please, please, don't hang up on me. We have to talk right now. Please…"

She was quite distraught. I sighed.

"Look Kathy, I'm sure you need to talk, but I don't think I want to listen to anything you have to say. And quite frankly, I have nothing to say to you." I rolled my tear-filled eyes. "I'm really angry with you right now. I mean, you've probably ruined both our lives, not to mention the possibility of getting us killed. Why in the world did you do this?" I asked despite knowing no explanation would be good enough.

"Jenny, I had no idea what was happening. They, actually, old Doc Kenalog, asked me if I would like to make a few extra dollars helping out on some additional cases. He said that special handling was needed, and I said, 'Sure.' I needed the money. I thought it was just that—making extra money and helping some businesses from out of town. I swear to you, Jenny, that's all they told me. I had no idea that it was going to be shady. I'm in as much danger as you are."

She sounded desperate. Kathy was often care-free, impractical every now and then, but never desperate. I started feeling sorry for her, but wasn't willing to end my grudge just yet.

"Yeah, well, why did you involve me in your money-making scheme? Why did you bet me to meet with those guys at the diner? Did you suspect it was going to be dangerous and you just decided you'd throw me to the wolves?"

"What? No!! It was nothing like that," Kathy shouted. "Jenny, you are always such a stick-in-the-mud with all your reading and working. The bet was actually more of a dare. It was completely innocent at the time. I knew that if I bet you to go meet with them, that you'd do it. I had no idea that it would be dangerous. I just thought you'd go meet them, get the details about the job, and we'd both earn a little extra money for what I thought was innocent work...I didn't know." Kathy stifled a sob. "I am so scared, Jenny," she whispered.

"Just shut up, Kathy, okay? Just shut up!" I didn't like to hear her this way. "I'm sure we can figure out a logical explanation for everything that's going on." *We can?* I doubted myself, but one of us had to be level headed. "Listen, why don't you come on over here? We'll go for a bike ride to clear our heads. Maybe being in a different environment will help us put things into perspective."

"All right, Jenny, I'll be over as soon as I can." Kathy sighed with relief.

After I put the phone on the cradle, I walked back to the window to watch the joggers and the children playing in the park. The birds were singing, and the world seemed to be a beautiful place. I assumed my leisurely Saturday morning routine wasn't in the cards for today.

I went back to the bathroom and unraveled my hair knowing it was going to be a lost cause since it was probably already dry. I hoped a quick flat-ironing and a few squirts of hairspray would help me to look presentable, at best. A knock at the door caused me to jump. I caught a glimpse of my haggard image in the hall mirror as I opened the door.

"Hi Kathy, come in. Do you want some coffee before we go?" I offered, letting bygones be bygones.

"No, I've had enough. Thanks anyway." Kathy smiled as she stepped inside. "I can't sleep at night now for fear that someone is going to snatch me at any minute. Let's see, they can take my liver and sell it for a couple thousand or maybe my..."

I stopped her in her tracks.

"Stop it, Kathy! Please turn off the dramatics. You're the one who got us into this bloody mess; now help me figure out what we need to do to get out of it. I don't want to hear another word about what they can sell or how much they can get for your organs!"

Kathy looked down at her shoes like a little child, obviously embarrassed by her behavior.

"Look," I continued, "I didn't mean to yell at you, but you've got to pull yourself together and help me, or we may be next. Let's just go for a bike ride and relax a little. Maybe we can get our ideas together."

Kathy looked up at me through those long eyelashes again and shrugged her shoulders. She knew I was right about this. I switched off the coffee pot, grabbed my keys, and locked the door on the way out.

CHAPTER SIX

The sun was shining on the sidewalk, casting shadows through the trees. Children were running in the park and having a wonderful time. How this evil thing could be happening in this lovely, wholesome town, I had no idea.

Kathy and I headed across the street to the rental place. We had been renting bikes for the past year because neither of us had the room in our apartments for a bicycle. We got our bikes and headed out on the bike trail as others rode past, laughing and yelling back and forth. The ride was pleasant. We rode in silence while admiring the sights on the trail. Flowers adorned both sides and appeared to greet us with enthusiasm as we passed. Up ahead we noticed a man with a pair of binoculars sitting on a bench. Kathy snapped her fingers to get my attention.

"Jenny, look at that man with the binoculars. Does he look familiar to you?" she whispered.

I saw who she was referring to and instantly felt a knot in my stomach.

"No. What is he looking at out here? And why would anyone come here wearing a suit and then sit on a park bench with a pair of binoculars?"

As we got closer to him, he turned the binoculars on us. Kathy became so startled, she ran into me with her bike, causing us both to tumble to the ground. The man in the suit quickly came running to where we landed in a heap on the trail.

His piercing eyes met ours. We were petrified. When he reached us, he leaned over to take my hand. As he attempted to pull me up, something slid from his coat pocket and fell into my lap. I screamed, but then realized it was just a book. I saw the title in big bold letters, "Bird Watching Because." I let out a sigh of relief. When I looked over at Kathy, she was as pale as a ghost. The man reached out and took Kathy's hand as well. He helped us pick up our bikes and asked if we were okay.

"Yes, I think that we're fine. Kathy, are you okay?" I asked.

"Yes, thank you, I'm okay," Kathy replied with an innocent smile.

"My name is John. I'm a bird enthusiast. When the weather is nice, I come out here during my lunch break to watch the birds."

He tilted his head and shrugged as I handed him back his book.

"Working on a Saturday, huh?" I eyed him suspiciously.

Before he had the chance to respond, Kathy hopped back on her bike and called out, "Thank you so much, sir, for helping us. I'm sorry that we disturbed you. Have a good day."

He waved to her as he walked back to the park bench. He sat down and resumed bird watching. I climbed back onto my bike, which seemed to be unharmed and continued down the trail after Kathy. I could tell this was all getting to be a bit too much for her. As we neared the end of the trail, we decided to stop and rest beside a babbling brook. We parked our bikes beside the others in the racks. Neither of us said a word. When we reached the picnic area, we sat down at a table and stared out over the crystal blue water. After a few quiet minutes, Kathy finally said what had been on her mind.

"Jenny, I am so sorry for getting you involved in this. If I had only known what was going on, I would not…I would … I… I'm so sorry." She buried her face into her hands.

"Kathy, it's okay." I patted her on the back. "I forgive you, and I know that you didn't know what was really going on. Let's just pull ourselves together and get this thing figured out, so we can get out of this situation alive. We know that Dr. Kenalog must be involved. He has participated in all of the hospital's donor retrieval cases."

Kathy wiped her eyes and nodded her head in agreement. I concentrated on what we knew so far and continued with my debriefing—both for her benefit and mine.

"I know the new girl must also be in on this because Dr. Kenalog called her in from New York. And guess what? Her parents own everything needed to run a tidy black market organ donation business. You know how there are drug rings and car theft rings? Maybe there are body theft rings, too. They own a funeral home, lab, and even a crematorium— perfect businesses for stealing and selling body parts. Don't you think?"

"I see what you mean, I think," Kathy said.

"Kathy, how can you be so naïve about this? What does it take for you to see what's going on here? Are you blind? Open your eyes. Pay attention. There are people being killed in strange accidents and did you hear about the prison breaks? And then there have been all of these extra flights in and out of town that no one has even questioned."

I shook my head trying to put together the pieces of the puzzle. Kathy nervously picked at her nails.

"How did you find out the new girl is involved?" she asked.

"Because, Kathy, I ran into her at the grocery store. She introduced herself then told me about her parents' businesses in New York. Her family is in a position to make all of the arrangements for The Code Blue Search Group. They can take the organs from the hospital, ship them all over the world and do whatever they're doing with them."

All of a sudden, a lightbulb went off in Kathy's head.

"Let's quit our jobs and leave! We can move to a bigger town and get good paying jobs at a bigger hospital. I'll pay half the rent on an apartment. We'd be better off leaving."

She was as enthused as a puppy ready to chase after a ball. Unfortunately, I felt it was my duty to rein her back in.

"No, Kathy, I'm sorry, but I'm not going to let them run us out of town. We're not moving or running from anything. We're going to stay here and solve this thing if it's the last thing we do, but I'm going to need your help. Are you with me, Kathy?"

Kathy knew it was the right thing to do since she was the one who got us into this mess. We needed to tackle this problem together. She took a deep breath and accepted her defeat.

"Yes," she replied, "I'm with you."

I reached out to clasp her hands in mine as a sign of our unified front. In doing so, I glanced at my watch and saw that it was getting late. It turned out to be a very pleasant day for both of us. It allotted us time to bond again. I had been hard on Kathy. Nerves were raw on both sides.

We walked back toward the bike rack. Once there, we discovered our bikes were gone. There was panic in Kathy's eyes and probably mine, too. Darkness would fall in an hour or so. It would take us at least thirty minutes to walk back to the rental shack.

"What are we going to do? Do you have your cell phone?" Kathy asked in tizzy.

"No, I left it at home so the hospital couldn't call us to come in today. We needed time to think. Calm down. Let's just start walking back. We'll look for the bikes along the way. Somebody probably took them by accident or maybe someone is trying to be cute. More than likely, it was just some kids playing a joke." I was trying to act unfazed, for her sanity's sake.

We walked at a fast pace. Up ahead on the right side of the trail, the bushes moved. Kathy saw it at the same time I did. She screeched, grabbed my arm, jerked me back, and then almost pulled me down to the ground.

"Who's there?" I called out.

Our feet were frozen in place. The rustling grew louder. Suddenly, a mama deer darted out of the bushes in front of us with her baby trotting right behind. Kathy was almost in tears and I wasn't far behind her. As they crossed to the other side of the woods, we both let out our breath that we were holding in unison.

"Phew!" I relaxed. "All right, let's try and settle down. We're okay. We're going to have a nervous breakdown if we don't try to lighten up a bit. Okay?"

"Okay," Kathy agreed.

All of the other bikers were long gone, and it was getting dark. We needed to hurry, so we started jogging. As we neared the bench where the bird watcher had been sitting, we saw no sign of our bikes. The rental shack wasn't too far. Just ahead we saw lights blinking, which gave us some comfort. Lights meant safety and the probability of human contact. There were no customers at the bike rental place. The guy working the booth just stared at us as we walked toward him.

"Okay, ladies, I hope you had a great ride, relaxed a little, and solved the problems of the whole working world ... like fixing it so no one will work but three days a week....right?" He seemed unconcerned that we were without bikes. "Here's your receipt, please do this again real soon. You owe me for a couple of hours, and then you're good to go." He handed a slip of paper to Kathy.

"How can we owe for only a couple of hours when we've had the bikes out all afternoon? And if you haven't noticed, we don't have the bikes. Someone stole them from us," I said, noting the obvious.

"Well, actually miss, your boyfriends brought back the bikes over an hour ago. All is fine. Actually, they said you ladies wanted to walk back, so ... oh yeah, and they left you a note. I almost forgot." He reached behind the counter for the folded yellow sticky note. "Here," he said as he handed me the note.

I looked at Kathy then hesitantly reached for the note. We paid the rental guy and thanked him. We didn't need anyone else in danger, so I didn't want to read the note in front of him. I didn't have to say that, but by the way Kathy pulled me across the street, she was thinking the same thing. Once we arrived in front of my apartment building, I couldn't wait any longer. I opened the note slowly. The words were written in dark blue ink. I read them aloud, "THE GROUP IS WATCHING YOU."

The blood drained from my face down to the soles of my feet.

Kathy was in a state of shock. They *were* following us!

Whoever they were, they could have been hiding behind any bush along the path at the park. And now, they were mocking us with this note! We entered the building in time to catch a glimpse of a wraithlike figure exiting the darkened stairwell. A plastic bag hung on my door knob. It seemed like an eternity before my hands would allow me to reach for it.

"Do you ... do ... I can get it, Jenny," Kathy stuttered.

"No, I'll do it."

I reached toward it with a fear that clutched at my throat as if someone were choking me. It was as if I was about to be attacked from the inside out. I held my breath as I took a look. I caught a glimpse of the book and eased it out of the bag. It took all my strength to open it as I read aloud the familiar title, "Bird Watching Because."

Kathy gasped and grabbed my arm. *I knew it! Nobody wears a suit on a Saturday!* I carefully cracked open the cover and read the bold print: "THE CODE BLUE SEARCH GROUP—STILL WATCHING YOU!"

I could feel my heart pounding all the way up to my ears. Neither of us could speak a word.

I dropped the keys to the door as sickness swept over me. I pulled myself together for a moment, and then exhaled before bending over to pick up the keys. I unlocked the door and we rushed into the apartment.

Before I had the chance to turn and lock the door behind us, a deep voice accosted us from the shadows of the living room....

"Hello, ladies! Glad you finally made it home from your little bike ride."

CHAPTER SEVEN

Kathy and I jumped out of our skin. We were both trembling. The two men I met at the diner were sitting in my living room as comfortably as if they were hanging out in their own homes. Without warning, something inside me just snapped.

"You have no right breaking into my apartment! How dare you?" Kathy held me back from my lunge.

"Why, Jenny, we have the key. We didn't need to break into your apartment. See?" He dangled my house key in the air like a dog treat.

This taunt was coming from the man who never said a word at the diner. I supposed I had been wrong to think he was mute.

"How did you get that?" I angrily grabbed at the air while Kathy kept her hold on me.

"We have our ways," responded Mr. Dark Eyes. He stood up from the couch and continued to speak as he walked around my living room, casually absorbing every inch of it. "Now, the reason for our little visit is to remind you and Miss Kathy here about a few things that we discussed during our first meeting." He ran his fingers along the back of my sofa and then quickly turned to look at us. "This is a private group. A *very* private group. You don't need to be questioning the other surgical team members at the hospital. We aren't too fond of your snooping. You'll be told everything you need to know, when you need to know it."

The man holding my key added, "Take our advice. Button your lips, or else. Do you understand what we're saying here?"

Kathy and I didn't respond. I stopped struggling and stood still. Kathy did not move a muscle. I was seething, but at the same time, I was petrified. "We really don't wish to demonstrate what could happen if you don't follow our orders."

He examined a framed photo of my parents that was displayed on the corner of my mantle. My nerves jolted up my spine and tension filled the air. He looked back at me and smirked. The look on my face surely gave it away. *Leave my parents out of this!* I was shouting on the inside. The evil man discovered my weakness and used it to his advantage. He fixed the buttons on his suit and continued with his threats.

"We hope we won't have to talk with your families. Although, we have been known to enjoy the little family talks and visits from time to time…if you girls get my drift."

Mr. Dark Eyes smiled while his partner laughed like a hyena. It was obvious they were enjoying their jobs. Kathy finally got up the nerve to respond.

"You had no right to break in here! No right at all! I'll call the sheriff on you two." She grabbed the phone from the end table and started to dial.

Mr. Dark Eyes sat down again, crossed his legs in a relaxed manner and replied, "Why, that's a really good idea Kathy. I think that would be Sheriff

Rodger Watson. Yep, old Uncle Rodge. He's a good ol' boy."

"What? You've got the sheriff working with you too?" Kathy hung up the phone.

"Well, I don't know if you can say he's working *with* us, as much as you might say he works *for* us. Made to look like he's been in charge in old morgue town for as long as I can remember...Yep, that's what we like to call it these days, Old morgue town. I'm sure you both understand that one!"

The hyena laughed again. Mr. Dark Eyes got up from the couch, shot a snide look at his partner who quieted his laugh and rose to his feet as well.

"Okay, ladies. All good things must end, so we're leaving. We'll let ourselves out." He seemed pleased with the round of torment that he just dished out.

The pair walked to the door unceremoniously, just like they did the first time I had seen them.

"Oh," the partner stopped, turned to face us and smiled as he added, "and thanks for the ham sandwiches. Good day!"

They slammed the door behind them. My legs felt like they would collapse underneath me. Kathy was sobbing. We hugged and tried to console each other.

The sheriff of Morganville was in on the whole thing. No one was safe. We had no idea who we could trust, if anyone. We didn't know who was a part of "The Group." Helplessness washed over me in waves. They already knew our daily routine, our family's goings and comings and every detail of our family's activities. I was so preoccupied in all of this that Kathy had slipped my mind. She stopped sobbing and sat on the couch to stare blankly into space. I got down on my knees to speak to her. She was in a fragile state.

"Please spend the night here with me, Kathy. Tomorrow is Sunday; we probably won't be called into the hospital. We can get up early in the morning and go for a drive in the country."

Her eyes were puffy from crying. She looked exhausted.

"We're fenced in, Jenny. We have no way of escape. We have no idea who is doing what. Maybe we'll be next if they think we've talked or done the wrong thing … maybe we…" She buried her face in her hands.

I took her hands into mine and tried to reassure her.

"Shhhh, look, why don't you take a shower? I'll make us a cup of hot chocolate, and we'll sit down and do nothing. We're beyond thinking rationally right now. Let's just chill."

Kathy paused and then nodded.

"Okay, Jenny, okay…okay. Yes, I will take it now … the shower I mean… if you say so."

While Kathy took her shower, I walked over to the window. Water for the hot chocolate was heating. As I looked out toward the park, the whole scene was one of serenity. The lights were dim, producing a glow that made the park look like a miniature fairy land.

I jumped when the teapot began to whistle. In the kitchen, I retrieved two cups from the upper cabinet. I poured the hot water into the cups and then I decided to add some liquor in with the chocolate. Maybe it would help us sleep. Kathy entered the kitchen as I placed the steaming cups on the kitchen table.

"Here, sit down and relax. The hot chocolate is mixed with a hint of liqueur; a little toddy for the body." I forced a smile.

My mind was racing in too many directions. *How could I possibly keep her calm during the days ahead when we were already on edge?* This town had its own rules now, made by players who had no faces or names. It seemed that most of the town was probably involved with The Group. We didn't have any real way of finding out the complete details of the situation until we got the final call that would explain it all. Neither of us knew when that would be. Kathy wasn't as strong as she appeared to be in the past. We sat sipping our hot chocolate in dead silence. What was left to say?

CHAPTER EIGHT

A few days had passed since our run in with The Group's goons. Kathy and I tried to act as though nothing was going on. We worked when we were supposed to, ate dinner together at my place, and crashed at night from the exhaustion brought on by the culmination of events. Though neither of us said anything, I was sure we were both hoping the nightmare would end on its own. It would have been nice to go on with our lives and forget about this whole thing.

Kathy and I finished doing the dishes and sat down to watch TV. Kathy was in no hurry to move back into her apartment. Though things seemed like they were getting back to normal, I think we were both enjoying each other's company and we felt safer staying together. Kathy was in a much better mood— she was back to joking around and teasing me. I wanted to join in her revelry, but I wasn't ready to put my guard down yet.

"Hey, maybe we can go on the river boat cruise this weekend; have a few drinks, dance a little and just relax. What do you think of that, Jenny?"

"Sounds good to me," I replied.

I could tell she was pleasantly surprised. Ordinarily, that sort of stuff was not my thing and Kathy would have had to drag me with her, kicking and screaming. She was happy I didn't put up a fight for once.

We flipped through the channels looking for the weather report. I said I'd take the boat cruise, but I wanted to make sure the weather would agree with that decision. We made small talk about our plans for the weekend, our parents, and some of our nursing school days. We did not, however, say a word about our jobs. Just as we were watching the weather report, a news bulletin broke in.

"It has just been learned that Sheriff Rodger Watson has called for back-up. Several deputies, along with medical personnel, are needed to work a major accident on Highway 24. They're reporting several fatalities. All members of the donor team are to report immediately to the hospital. I repeat you are to report to the hospital immediately. The sheriff states the team members know who they are and what is expected of them."

My heart began to race as I looked over at Kathy. Her face was pale.

"Kathy, we are going to have to get ready. You know he'll be calling here. Just mark my words he'll be..."

At that moment, the phone rang out like a fire alarm.

"Get dressed, Kathy," I stated. "You know that's him. We can't get out of this."

I hesitated, then answered the phone.

"Hello?"

The familiar voice responded.

"Dr. Kenalog here. There's been a major accident on the highway. We need our best team members to get to the hospital immediately. After all, you are on call."

I frowned at his snide reminder.

"Yes doctor, we know about the accident. It was on the news. We'll be there right away, sir."

We dressed hurriedly for the emergency call. I wondered how Dr. Kenalog could possibly know that the people in the accident were organ donors. Why would they call out a team whose only involvement was organ donor retrievals? There were so many things that we couldn't answer. Nothing made sense. We decided to leave Kathy's car and head to the hospital in mine. I wasn't sure that I was in good enough condition mentally to drive, but someone had to get us there.

"Do you suppose Chloe will be there?" Kathy asked.

"Surely you are making a joke now, right?" I couldn't pretend that I was happy with the situation.

"No, I'm not being funny in the least," she responded defensively. "Maybe she gets to take off because of her dad's position at the hospital. It isn't such a far out idea, you know."

I rolled my eyes, shook my head, and didn't answer. Thankfully, Kathy kept quiet for the remainder of the ride.

I had worked at another hospital for ten years. Three of those years were spent with a donor team. We never had this many cases. The donor program was essential. Many people would have died without the gift of life from someone willing to become a donor. So many patients needed kidneys, livers, and skin grafts. There were groups of wonderful donor programs across the country. During the years I worked with that program, the hospital made sure that we learned all about the paperwork and how to assure safe donor matches. Safety measures were critical from beginning to end, and there were strict demands that the staff follow the protocols. Everything worked together to guarantee that procedures were properly carried out for all involved, including the deceased.

Kathy had previously worked in a donor program for six months, but she really never knew about the mechanics involved. She sat rigid as we drove to the hospital. Time seemed to fly by, and before we wanted to be, we were there. We pulled into the parking lot and headed to the closest parking space. We spotted a black Hummer with New York tags as I parked my car. The vehicle was conspicuous in a small town hospital parking lot.

"Do you see that?" Kathy was referring to the out-of-place vehicle. "Look at the tags. That car reeks of money. I wonder if it belongs to Chloe's parents. Who else would have a car like that in Morganville?"

Well, I don't think it is Chloe's car because I didn't see it when I ran into her at the store.

A car like that would have been pretty obvious."

"Look, there goes Chloe." I pointed her out while holding Kathy back at the hospital entrance. "She's about to get on the elevator. Let's wait a sec and let her go up ahead of us. I don't want to talk to her now."

We waited a few moments giving Chloe time to get off on the next floor. Then we got on the elevator. As we stepped off, we noticed Chloe talking to a man who was standing with Dr. Kenalog. We didn't know the identity of the man, but Kathy and I recognized him as Dr. Kenalog's assistant in the case we worked the day before. Chloe was quite friendly with the man. All three looked toward us as we headed in their direction. We turned into the nurses' lounge and started changing into our scrubs when Chloe walked in the room.

"Hey, Jenny, Kathy. How's it going these days? You guys know that we have got to hurry. We'll be in trouble if we're late. We have three rooms ready and waiting. The docs are antsy to get on with the slicing and dicing ... oops, sorry, just making a funny." She giggled and shrugged as she checked her teeth in the mirror.

She turned and headed toward the main operating room, leaving Kathy and me standing there with our painted-on smiles.

We were in another world now. We seemed to be fumbling at things that had become routine in our careers.

"Where do we go, Jenny? What do we do? There have never been three operating rooms full of donors before. No one has told us anything. And Chloe ... she is so smug and..." Panicky Kathy was back.

"Ladies, may I inquire as to why you aren't already in there getting the back tables ready and the patient draped and prepped for this procedure?" Dr. Kenalog asked gruffly. "You two are standing here talking as if you have nothing to do. What's your problem?"

We both stared at him blankly. Someone we didn't know was with Dr. Kenalog. His name tag read Dr. Evans. Kathy broke the silence.

"Dr. Kenalog, sir, we just got here and our.... uh, we are.... well, where do you want us to go, sir?"

"Jenny, you go to O.R. number three. Kathy, you go to number two. You'll be working with a new doctor, Dr. John Evans." He gestured to the man standing next to him. "Dr. Evans, this is Kathy. She will be assisting you today. By the way, Kathy and her friend are two of the best in the field. That's why we have tapped into their services. They will fit in quite nicely when the time is right, if you know what I mean."

Dr. Kenalog ribbed Dr. Evans while he shook his head approvingly.

"Dr. Evans is visiting from New York and will be assisting me in all of my ongoing experiments and important matters for a long time to come. You need to get well acquainted with him and learn all of his work habits. Kathy, do you hear me?"

Kathy jumped to attention.

"Go to O.R. number two with Dr. Evans," he commanded.

"Yes, sir, Dr. Kenalog, I will, sir..." Kathy replied. "I was just wondering, Dr. Evans, is Chloe your daughter, sir?"

"Why yes, she is my daughter." Dr. Evans suddenly beamed with pride. "Actually, she is my right hand man, so to speak. You will be working with her more, too. Yes, you both will be seeing Chloe often."

I wondered why Kathy had been sent to work with a new doctor, but then that wasn't so hard to figure. She is not very suspicious or doubtful of others, but I am. She isn't too perceptive at times either, unless a specific medical procedure is involved.

Dr. Kenalog turned to look at me. He nodded as a signal for me to follow him into O.R. number three. I followed him and said nothing. I walked in expecting to see Chloe, but she wasn't there. A group of unfamiliar faces met my gaze as we walked over to the cadaver, which had already been prepared.

Dr. Kenalog walked around the table and mumbled something to the taller guy at the head of the table. The guy nodded and indicated that he understood. The body remained covered.

"Jenny, go to the back table," Dr. Kenalog directed. "Get the preservatives ready and the containers labeled. We'll be taking kidneys, lymph tissue, and skin. Get everything ready for quick transport. The sheriff will have a car and driver here to pick up the specimens in four hours."

"Doctor, I don't think…I… there are no permit papers here, nothing for me to fill out and check…" I regretted the words as soon as they came out of my mouth.

"Jenny, I think I told you the last time, I will take care of the paperwork. You are not to concern yourself with that. Do you understand?"

"Yes, sir, I think I fully understand." I looked down at my shoes wishing for an escape route.

"And exactly what does that remark mean? What are you trying to say to me in that snippy tone of yours?" he asked.

"Nothing, Dr. Kenalog," I muttered. "I'm sorry. I'll get things ready, sir."

I quickly returned to the back table. I tried to keep my trembling hands busy.

Dr. Kenalog went through the procedure with the help of his assistants.

We finished the case, and I completed the labeling of the containers. Dr. Kenalog told me to leave; he would complete the closure of the body. I knew what that meant: he wanted me out of his way. As I walked out the door, I saw Sheriff Watson. I knew he was here to pick up and transport the tissue collections, although I was told a driver would be sent. What difference did it make anyway? We all had a role in this illegal activity. I had never seen the variation of cases that I was seeing now. God help us all!

CHAPTER NINE

Kathy and I rode the elevator down in silence. Kathy looked extremely pale. There wasn't a need to question her while on the hospital premises. Others got on the elevator making small talk about patients, kids and trivial matters of the day. It was a shift change. People were coming and going in a rush. We made a beeline to my car.

"Look, Dr. Evans is still here," Kathy said.

We both stared at the Hummer with the New York license plate.

"Hurry, let's get out of here," I replied.

We looked all around us before jumping into my car. No one was in sight as far as we could tell.

"What's wrong Kathy? You look as pale as a ghost. What happened today with the new doc?"

"Weird things happened; crazy, weird stuff!" Kathy exclaimed.

"What do you mean?" I wondered. *What could be crazier than stealing organs?*

"Well, first of all, the back table wasn't set up. The body was a young man in his thirties. He was admitted to the hospital for some kind of minor surgery. I swear to you, he was breathing the whole time. His chest rose and fell. It was shallow, but I could see it! The others accused me of imagining things.

His cause of death was listed as a blood clot. He was hooked up to the IV, and…I just think I…"

"What did Dr. Evans say about all of this?" I asked.

"He just kept telling me that he didn't have time for such an absurd conversation. Then he sent me down to the supply room, telling me that he needed supplies from CSR."

"CSR? Did you go?" I couldn't understand what she was talking about. Maybe she was hallucinating.

"Yes, of course I did what he asked of me. Are you crazy enough to think that I could say no to him? What should I have said? 'Well doc, let me think about this because seeing what the blue blazes ya'll are doing to this man, who is obviously very much alive, is more important than me going to the CSR right now!'"

"You're nuts, Kathy! You've stepped over the boundaries. You can't even talk to me rationally about your observations. Nothing you're telling me makes a bit of sense." I hit my hand against the steering wheel to let out some of my frustration. "Personally, I think you've flipped your lid! What did he make you get from CSR anyway? I mean, what could he have been doing to the man that would've required more equipment?"

"He told me to get another neuro set-up plus the newest type of head tongs."

"What for? No one has ever attempted to use those tongs. The docs always prefer using the old standby equipment. It's funny how they will order from smooth talking reps just to get favors."

"I don't know, Jenny, it's strange, and then we see all of the unethical practices being treated as mundane occurrences. Dr. Evans said they were keeping him hydrated until something about legal papers and issues with his wife were worked out. I don't know what eventually happened since the doctor asked me to leave the O.R."

"You sound like...just never mind. Something tells me that you've lost your perspective in this thing! You need a break. I mean, how could you be in there and not observe some of what went on in that room? You're making no sense, Kathy. Where was the body when you went back in there?"

"There wasn't a chance of me going back in there," Kathy replied. "He called CSR himself and told them to send what he needed up on the dumbwaiter. He insisted that home was the best place for me. I didn't do a thing today except go to CSR. I think...well...it's like he wanted me to be there as a witness in some way to help him out, as an alibi or something. I don't know; it's just a hunch."

We drove in silence the remainder of the way. The only sounds we heard were of people honking horns. They were all in a hurry to get nowhere. I knew in my mind that she was right. Something wasn't kosher. Maybe he wanted Kathy there as an alibi for whatever he had planned. That way, he couldn't be blamed for anything in the future. Kathy couldn't say he did anything wrong if she hadn't witnessed him doing anything wrong. Oh, he was clever all right, and his story was far from being unraveled. It crossed my mind that Kathy was in more danger than I was. I hoped I was wrong, but at any rate, I wouldn't say a thing to her. She was already a basket case.

As we neared the apartment, we saw the flashing red lights of several ambulances and fire trucks. They were in the park across the street. The streets were crowded. People were crying and running in all directions. The police officers had the sidewalk and the street in front of my apartment roped off. There wasn't any way to get to my parking space.

We parked about a block away and walked back to the roped-off area. I hoped that being dressed in our nursing uniforms would get us close to the action so we could find out what was going on.

"What do we do if the paramedics have it under control?" Kathy asked. "They might not let us inside the area, and we'll never know what..."

"Well, now, if it isn't Miss Jenny and Miss Kathy all geared up for their Florence Nightingale adventures! How are you two girls doing on this sultry night?" asked the man in the uniform.

"Uh, Sheriff Watson, we just left the hospital and were headed to my apartment. I live..."

"Girly, where you live is not a secret in the least." The officer snorted and puffed out his chest. "That's the business of the sheriff's office and the sheriff. I know all about you and Kathy here. Now, you girls can go on to your apartment. Clearance for you will be arranged."

"But, Sheriff, we thought maybe we could help out with whatever is going on and..." Kathy tried to volunteer our services, but Sheriff Watson wasn't interested.

"Well, now, that is right kind of you ladies, but things are under control. Everything is almost finished. We're getting ready to move outta here in a few more minutes. You ladies go to your apartment, now. I said I'll get you clearance," he replied, more assertively this time. He lifted the police tape that roped off the area and waved us through.

"Yes, sir. Thank you," I said. "Let's go, Kathy. We've had a long day. We'll fix a snack, and you can spend the night again."

I led the way while Kathy followed close behind me. There was still a lot of commotion, but there was no way to tell what was going on without veering off the path. I assumed the sheriff was watching us, so we continued until we arrived at my apartment building.

"Are you sure you want me to stay?" Kathy asked once we were safely out of earshot. "I mean, I've been here for several days already Jenny. I know how much you cherish your space."

"Yes, of course I want you to stay," I replied, surprising even myself. Kathy was right.

I did enjoy my alone time, but with everything that was going on, we were safer to stay together.

"Oh, what are we going to do, Jenny? Maybe we should pack up and move to another town or something?"

I stopped in front of my door to answer her.

"Kathy, we've discussed this numerous times. We are not running from this. The plan is to stay here and fight until their end or ours, if that be the case. We've done nothing wrong. Now, let's go make a cup of tea and grab a sandwich."

I unlocked the door and we quickly entered the apartment. A pact had been made between us that we would never go in again without checking around first. I no longer felt safe since those men had come into my apartment. We flipped the light switches in each of the rooms. Everything looked clear.

We put together sandwiches and ate in silence. Kathy got up to help me clear the table, but I took the plates from her and brought them to the sink. I hoped that by washing the dishes I could have a few minutes to myself to organize my thoughts.

"Why don't you get comfortable, and turn on the news. Maybe we can see what happened in the park since Sheriff Watson refused to tell us," I suggested.

"Yes, maybe, but I'm not so sure that I even want to know. Do you?"

Kathy hesitated with the remote in her hand.

"Well, yes, I do. For Pete's sake Kathy, it is just across the street. It's one of those *need* to know things." *Ignorance is NOT bliss!* I yelled at her in my mind.

I grabbed the remote from her hands, turned the television on, and then dropped the remote in her lap. I went back to the dishes as Kathy flipped through the channels until she got to the news station. They were just finishing up the story on what was happening in the park.

"At this time, we don't know the cause of death. The police will notify the next of kin before releasing the identity of the deceased to the public. This wraps up this portion of the evening news." The news anchor then signed off for the night.

"Jenny, we missed it. They said there was another dead body right across from your apartment. Aren't you scared?"

I stood in the doorway to the living room drying my hands.

"Yes, of course I am. But you know me; I feel the need to be prepared as well. A gun permit is the next step. I'll keep a loaded gun in my bedside table from now on. Do you have a gun?"

I asked as nonchalantly as if I were asking whether or not she liked sugar in her tea.

"A gun? No! Of course not!" Kathy straightened up on the couch and folded her feet underneath her. "And even if I did, I don't know how to shoot!"

"Well, you're going to learn." I sounded like her parent. "Tomorrow we'll go to the gun shop. We should each buy a small caliber hand gun and get the necessary permits to carry them. That will make us both feel safer for now." I wasn't sure if I was trying to convince her or myself.

"Alright," Kathy answered, "I don't like the idea of such a thing, but this is not the time for bickering over my beliefs about killing, I suppose."

I picked up the remote and turned off the television. We didn't need to hear anymore bad news.

"Okay, let's go to bed. We have an early day tomorrow, and it's going to be hectic. Set your clock, so we won't be late. Mine is on the blink again." I yawned.

"No problem." Kathy yawned back at me. "Oh, and after work tomorrow, I'll need to go back to my place to pick up some more clothes. How long do you want me to stay here?"

"Maybe we should just play it by ear. I think it's much safer for both of us this way.

Unless you just want to wait until you are comfortable using a gun."

I wasn't sure if that was ever going to happen, but I didn't want her to be afraid of what might be our only form of protection.

"Actually, I don't really want to be alone, Jenny, no more than you do." She assumed correctly. "We can share expenses if you don't mind and I'll bring over enough clothes for a few weeks, if that's okay with you."

"That sounds good." I nodded and headed to my bedroom. "Night, Kathy."

"Night, Jenny."

As I passed my bedroom window, I caught a glimpse of the swirling lights from the ambulance. A couple of police cars were still outside. The lights seemed to shout out silent warnings. Things were getting out of hand. I eased myself under my comforter and finally allowed my eyes to rest. A sudden rap at the door caused me to scream.

"What's wrong with you, Jenny? Why did you scream? Is someone in your room?" Kathy called out in a panic.

"You scared the life out of me! What do you want?" I growled with my heart still outside of my chest.

"You said for me to set the bloody clock. There isn't a clock in the room. Don't you get huffy with me, especially now."

"Next time you ought to..." I peeled back my covers in a huff and grabbed the old alarm clock from my bottom drawer.

"Ought to what? Huh?" Kathy was still instigating from the other side of my door.

I opened the door quickly and she jumped back.

"Nothing," I answered. "Here, take the clock." I shoved it into her chest. "And go to bed!" I shut the door in her face.

We were both on edge, and of course, we were tired. I got back into bed assuming that Kathy would forgive my rude behavior eventually. I lay there in the dark as the lights continued to play their helical games on the ceiling. It was not a playground of dreams conducive to sleep. I lay there for what seemed like an eternity before my eyes became heavy again. Finally, I fell into a deep sleep.

CHAPTER TEN

"Jenny, get up!" Kathy shouted while pounding on my bedroom door. "I'm sorry I overslept. Jenny! The clock went off, but I went back to sleep. Jenny! Wake up!"

"Okay, okay. I hear you!" I shouted back. "Now stop yelling before the neighbors call the law!"

The pounding ceased. As I climbed out of bed and staggered to the bathroom, I was hoping that Kathy would make the coffee. The shower felt relaxing, but since we were running late, I couldn't allow myself this luxury for very long. The smell of fresh-brewed coffee drifted into my nostrils. *Ahhhh!* I grinned. I went into the kitchen and poured myself a cup. The window attracted me like a moth to a flame. It was a 'Sunday morning' kind of view, like looking at a place of serenity. It didn't look like yesterday's death scene. I was curious about what really happened in the park.

"Why are you staring out the window? What's wrong now?" Kathy asked.

"Oh, good morning, Kathy. There's nothing wrong. I was just looking at the park and the normalcy of the day. It's so hard to believe that a dead body was in that beautiful setting last night." I took a sip of my coffee.

"Are you going to get ready to go or are you just going to stare out of the window all day?"

Jeez! Either somebody woke up on the wrong side of the bed this morning or she's still mad at me for slamming the door in her face last night. Oh well. It serves her right for scaring the heck out of me.

Without turning to face her, I answered sweetly, "It won't take me long, Kathy; just a few minutes. I've already fixed my hair."

Kathy smirked but resisted the urge to comment. I quickly got dressed. Moments later we grabbed our purses and headed out. Since we didn't want to go to work, the drive seemed unusually short. We found a place to park. Chloe was coming toward us from across the parking lot. She was speaking so fast; it was hard to keep up with all the information.

"Hi, Jenny. Kathy. Are ya'll ready for the big day? Daddy says it'll be busy today. Just last night he commented to someone on the phone that Morganville had become a bustling little town. You know that young guy we worked with yesterday had to be kept on hydration therapy. They sent him to another room to do a particular procedure, and…oh, I forgot that you were with Daddy during that case, Kathy. Daddy said you had to go to CSR. Well, we better hurry, girls. You know Daddy doesn't really like to be kept waiting."

We watched as she walked ahead of us. She was in a big hurry. I felt my skin crawl every time she was around. It was a foreboding feeling that came over me.

"What was that all about?" Kathy asked.

"How should I know?" I checked my reflection to make sure my hat was on securely. "I'm sure we'll find out soon enough."

We walked into the hospital. The elevator doors were open. We hurried to get on. It was full of people, as usual. We had already decided not to discuss what was going on while we were in the hospital. We stepped off in time to see a man pushing a body on a gurney into the empty room beside one of the operating rooms. No one had gone into that deserted room since a man was murdered there years ago.

They said he was a well-known doctor who had gotten strung out on drugs and alcohol. None of the staff was willing to discuss the details of what happened the night of the murder. I heard rumors that the doctor may have been hallucinating due to some of his actions before his death. It was a subject that remained taboo to speak about in the hospital.

It was very strange that the body was taken into that particular room, but I was not about to ask a soul. I looked at Kathy, and she looked at me. We said nothing. We walked over to look at the assignment sheet that was hanging beside the lounge. Kathy and I were going to be with Dr. Kenalog. Chloe was with her dad and a doctor whom neither of us recognized. We went in to scrub up and entered the operating room just in time to see the doctor inject the patient. Usually the recipient of the organ would be given an antibiotic. I had no clue what was happening. No one was following protocol in any way. Neither Kathy nor I said a word as we took our places beside the table.

"Okay, the family signed the paperwork for the organs. We'll start with getting the skin prepped and sterile. We will remove it first, and then move to all usable organs. We will take the eyes last," Dr. Kenalog explained for our benefit.

We looked at each other. There had never been total organ retrieval at the hospital before; we weren't sure of what to do.

"Jenny, get the prep kit." Dr. Kenalog pointed. "Kathy, go heavy with the Betadine on the skin. Let's go now!"

We followed the doctor's commands and finished the case within the hour. A separate container was set up, but it was not labeled. I mentioned that to the doctor and was given a stern look for an answer. From then on, I kept my mouth shut. He instructed Kathy to leave then excused himself as he turned away from me. I was also told to leave. When I left the room, I noticed that the lights were on in the closed-off room next door. Kathy was standing in the hall looking at the room, as well. We both knew we needed to get out of there as fast as possible, but we had to take a quick peek in the room. The windows were blocked with a thick black curtain. It was clear that they didn't want anyone snooping around.

I knew that neither Kathy nor I had any reason to look into what was going on in there, but I also knew we had to check it out anyway. There was something drawing us to that room.

"Watch out for me, Kathy. I'll see if anyone is in there. If not, then we can go in and look around, just for a second. Go over to the O.R. doors and watch the doctors in the first two rooms. The other rooms are dark, so hurry!"

Kathy scurried over to where the other procedures were still going on while I edged my way quietly to the curtained door. I eased the door open far enough to see two gowned figures standing over a body. They were deep in conversation. They didn't appear to see or hear me. There was no possible way of getting into the room as long as they were there. One of the figures turned to the side table and reached for an object in a container. It was so small that it was barely visible from the door. The other gowned figure made a small incision in the head of the body. Both figures leaned over the table intent on what they were doing. There was an IV hooked to the body containing what appeared to be normal saline or a similar fluid. I inched the door open a little more to get a better view of the room and the people inside.

"Jenny!" Kathy tapped me on the back.

I jumped and turned my head back to her.

"What the ... you scared the..."

"Jenny, we've got to hurry. Both rooms are closing their cases. The doctors will be coming out any moment. Let's get out of here now. Hurry, let's go!"

"Shh, be quiet. Hush or you'll get us killed right here!" I spoke as softly as I could while still expressing my anger.

"Well, if you don't come on now, I'll leave you standing here to pay the grim reaper. So, come on!" Kathy was insistent.

"All right, give me time to ease the stupid door shut." As I carefully and quietly eased the door closed, I felt the presence of a large figure looming behind me.

"Well now, what in the world do we have here? Peeping nurses? Hmm?"

We turned around and stared right into the angry faces of Dr. Kenalog and Dr. Evans. Both of them looked at us with eyes that could pierce the body like a stiletto.

"Well, sir, we heard noises and thought that something was wrong. And … and… this room is closed. And we just… just…We are leaving now, uh sir." Kathy tried to sound innocent while ushering me away from the door.

Doctor Kenalog leaned in over us. His hot breath spit out each of his words.

"I suggest that you ladies keep your noses out of places that they don't belong. Do you understand me?"

"Yes, Dr. Kenalog, we understand." I couldn't bear to look at him. I was too afraid. "We're leaving for home now. We didn't see anything in the room…Well, I mean there were two men and they were…uh…We are going, sir. We'll see you tomorrow." I nodded to Dr. Evans, then turned to my partner in crime. "Kathy, let's go."

As we ushered ourselves down the hallway, we could feel their eyes boring into our backs.

"You see Jenny! I told you we needed to go, and you just wouldn't listen. I'm so mad that you didn't move when I told you to."

"Shut up, Kathy! I know, but let's not walk around here bickering over this. We need to play dumb from now on until we get to the bottom of this thing. We have to alert the police about what we know."

Kathy stopped in her tracks.

"But we don't know who in the police department is or isn't in on this thing!"

"Would you hush!" I grabbed her arm and led her into the nurses' lounge. "That's the chance we're going to have to take."

We swiftly changed and got out of the hospital as fast as possible. Kathy and I were scared. There was something ominous going on in the closed off room. That room had been shut off for so long that no one even knew it was being used, or if they did know, they weren't talking about it.

My thoughts were scattered in all directions. *What was The Group doing with the organ shipments?* There were substantial financial gains to be made in illegal organ donations. I knew that there were many countries involved in the organ donor black market. It had made the news more than once. *Why would someone want or need the kind of money that would force them into illegal dealings, unethical practices, and forsaking the Hippocratic Oath? Where would all of this take us? Would we be the next victims?* I didn't know what to do; danger had settled around us.

CHAPTER ELEVEN

We were in the parking lot headed for the car. I didn't really want to take the chance of being overheard, so I didn't say anything.

"Jenny, what do we do?"

Kathy was nervously twirling her hair between her fingers. I pulled the keys out of my purse and stared her down.

"I'm going to unlock the doors, and we are going to get in the car. Then, I am going to forget what I saw today. You'd better do the same if you know what's good for you."

We scrambled into the car. When I sat down behind the wheel, I realized the seat had been moved as far back as it could go. Someone had broken into my car. I gasped.

"Someone has been in here, Kathy. Look, I can't even touch the gas pedal."

I adjusted my seat then turned the key in the ignition. The car made a grinding noise. I tried again. The engine was dead as a doornail. *Who did this?* I was angry. If the guards had been patrolling the parking lot like they were supposed to, this wouldn't have happened.

"What do we do now, Jenny? What are you going to do?" Kathy pulled at her seat belt, as if putting it on would save her life at this point.

"Kathy, for Pete's sake, please just stop it! The last thing I need is for you to get crazy on me."

I grabbed my cell phone and got out of the car. Somehow, I was able to open the hood. The battery was intact, but there were loose wires coming out in every direction. I had no clue what they were for or where they needed to be connected. Thank goodness I had a membership to a towing service. I felt my chest tighten as I dialed the number.

The parking lot was pretty quiet. Kathy was sitting in the front seat, crying and blowing her nose all at the same time. Hysteria was building up inside me as I ended the phone call. I started to laugh uncontrollably. However, nothing was going to be solved by acting like a fool. Surely someone was trailing our every move. We obviously had become their main target. They were probably watching us this very minute.

"Okay, the wrecker company said they will have a serviceman here in a few minutes. We'll be on our way to the apartment soon." Kathy looked at me like I had lost my mind. I paced beside the driver's side door and ranted. "The car will be fixed, and we will be fine. Just tell yourself that all is well."

A few minutes later, I looked up and saw the tow truck pulling up beside us. They had instructed me to leave the hood up, so they would be able to find us in the parking lot.

"Hey there, ma'am. You must be the little lady in need." The short, stout man greeted me as he jumped out of his truck.

"Yes, sir. We seem to have wire problems here." I pointed under the hood. "There are wires going in every direction. Could you tell me just by looking under here how this could have happened?"

"Well, now, let me take a gander at it while you put your John Hancock on this here paper saying that I did come fer a breakdown. Maybe I kin figure it out or I might not. Everything ain't a cut and dried deal, ya know?"

He smiled while offering me a clipboard with his greasy hands. I graciously accepted the paperwork, but ducked into my car to find a clean pen.

"All right, I see the problem as plain as the nose on an elephant's face," he called out from under the hood. "Yep, these here wires right over here were disconnected from the coil. All I gotta do is to hook her back up, and she's ready to roll. Okay, now you're ready to go. Crank 'er up."

I breathed a sigh of relief as the engine started up on my first try. Kathy and I rushed out to thank the tow truck driver. He gave us the thumbs up and dropped the hood closed.

"But how could this possibly happen, sir? I mean, did the wires just disconnect because I hit a curb or something?"

I waited for his expert opinion while handing back his clipboard.

"Nah, ma'am, nah, ain't no way on earth that'd done it. This here was done a 'purpose. Yep! Someone is mad at you, or you've got friends that have a banged up sense of humor." He wiped his hands on a dirty towel that hung from his pants pocket. "Yep, this is a planned job alright. Someone put the old magic marker on ya, ma'am. And I figger you girls must know who got your number too, don't cha?"

"No sir. Actually, we have no idea who did this to us," Kathy replied.

The tow truck driver was scratching his chin and giving us a strange, or maybe, a fearful look. I wasn't sure which it was.

"Hmm, well then, ya'll sure need to be careful out there. Yep, you sho nuff made some folks mad at you." He continued shaking his head like he was sorry to tell us this insight. Then, realizing his job was done, he patted on the hood of my car and waved us off. "Okay, ladies, she's ready to git a'rolling. Ya'll take care now."

We watched him leave the parking lot. His words were unsettling. Someone had tampered with the wires in an attempt to communicate a message to us; it definitely got our attention. It seemed like every minute there was a new mind game. But what was the game? Who was playing and why?

We got back into the car and sat silently for a moment.

"Who do you think did this?" Kathy asked. "Is someone going to kill us next? Jenny, why don't you talk to me and quit sitting there looking the way you are?"

I gripped the steering wheel with all my might and whipped my head towards her to respond.

"Do I look like a psychic to you, Kathy?"

Suddenly, we both burst out laughing, then crying, and then consoling each other. Fear was wreaking havoc on both of us causing emotional outbursts. We needed each other now more than ever. As I shifted the car into drive, we both looked around the parking lot. There didn't seem to be anyone watching us, or at least we couldn't see them if they were there.

After our pre-planned stop at the gun store, we drove to the apartment. I unlocked the door and we cautiously looked around. We were afraid of everything. Nothing looked out of the ordinary, so we walked inside. We should have called the sheriff about the car, but we figured it wouldn't matter to him. He was not going to get the satisfaction of knowing we were frightened, so we decided not to report the incident.

"We've had a busy day, Jenny. I am mentally and physically exhausted. Oh, did you see the schedule for tomorrow?"

"Yes. Chloe is floating in each of the rooms tomorrow.

She's going to be filling out the reports for the donor retrievals. What does that make you think?" I asked with raised eyebrows.

"Do you really think that Chloe and her dad are dishonest or just being snowed by Dr. Kenalog?" Kathy wondered.

Did she just not want to believe that people could be evil or was she just naive?

"They're not one bit ignorant. Open your eyes, Kathy, and use your head. They're not honest. They're too involved in every facet of the different programs. They stand to gain financially from all of this. No, they know exactly what is going on. Of that, I am sure. They're two sharp cookies. If you observe them in their actions, you will see that they have walked this road for a long time. They are very skilled in what they do."

"I know you're right. I suppose I was hoping for some professional honesty in this organization."

I need to stop being so hard on her, I reminded myself.

"Let's eat a sandwich and go to bed. I am disgusted and tired of thinking about all of it."

We went into the kitchen, made a cup of hot chocolate, and fixed our sandwiches. It was getting late. Neither one of us wanted to talk about it anymore. We finished our meal and went to our rooms. We were emotionally drained.

I tossed and turned all night. I had nightmares about body parts. The parts were all lined up for sale like cuts of meat at the supermarket. I woke up to the eerie glow of the clock. It was 3:45 a.m. The alarm clock was set for 5:00 a.m. I couldn't go back to sleep. Instead of lying in bed staring at the ceiling, I decided to get up. I wandered into the living room then peered out the window. The park was so beautiful and well kept. An array of blooming flowers surrounded the oak trees. A park that was the replica of something from Cape Cod should not be tainted by death.

Morganville was known for its tourist attractions. Of primary interest were the Craftsman-style bungalow homes where famous people from the eighteenth century had resided. There were rumors that other well-known gentlemen had lived in the town, including a famous poet. He supposedly lived in Morganville during the summer months with his mistress.

I turned around and saw Kathy standing behind me. She was staring out the window past me.

"What are you doing up, Kathy? Can't you sleep?"

"No," she answered rubbing her eye. "I had horrible nightmares about shadows dancing toward me and a group of faceless people dressed in long white robes. Sometimes I feel as if I'm losing my mind or something."

"I know the feeling. But, things will get better. One day we'll look back on this ordeal and be so grateful that we survived. Why, we'll make the hometown news when we crack this case and everything is out in the open and..." My wishful thinking was interrupted.

"Why is the phone ringing at this time of the morning?" Kathy eyed me with curiosity.

"I don't know."

I watched as Kathy walked over to pick it up, but then stopped herself.

"You get it, Jenny. It's your house." Kathy handed me the phone.

I answered the phone, but didn't even have a chance to say "Hello" before the ominous voice attacked me.

"Now listen very closely, Jenny. You and your friend better keep your noses out of my business. Do you understand me, Miss?"

I shook my head, but couldn't muster up a voice to reply. *How'd he know it was me on the phone?* I glanced out the window. *They must be using binoculars or something because I haven't said a word!* I pulled the blinds closed.

He continued, "Well, you better understand, because if you start snooping around again, both you and Kathy will be our next donors."

The phone fell from my hand. I held onto a chair as I made my way to the couch.

"What is it, Jenny? You look like you've seen a ghost. Tell me what's going on. Who was on the phone?" Kathy followed and sat down next to me.

"That was someone with The Group, and he said that if I, or we, didn't keep our noses out of his, or their, business, that we would be the next ones in the O.R."

"What are you saying?" Kathy looked puzzled.

"It means we will be the next donor cases. We've got to be extremely careful if we are going to continue spying. We've been caught, and they're angry."

I sat staring straight ahead. Kathy looked at me like she was waiting for me to provide her with words of wisdom, but I didn't have anything to give.

CHAPTER TWELVE

I snapped out of my daze and stood up from the couch.

"We need to keep level heads, Kathy. Let's get ready for work. It's almost time to go anyway. We can stop in the cafeteria and get a donut and coffee or something before we clock in."

Kathy headed to the shower. I went to my bedroom. The wheels started turning in my head as never before. We were ready to walk out the door when the phone rang again. It was Chloe. She said the first case had been cancelled. The next one was at eight-thirty. We would have plenty of time to focus before this morning's case. I thought we could bring this Code Blue Search Group out into the open. One of the ideas that went through my mind was to wear a wire. Managing such a thing would require plenty of rational planning, and Kathy probably wasn't going to go for it.

We headed to the car. The radio was set on an easy listening station. An oldie played in the background: Rod Stewart singing Maggie May, which was a favorite from my younger days. It took my mind back in time for a moment. Kathy and I attempted to make small talk. Neither one of us really wanted to deal with reality.

The parking lot at the hospital was unusually crowded. We had to drive around for a while before finding a place to park. The back lot was always empty, but we would have to take the shuttle bus from there. Neither one of us wanted to do that because it was too secluded and too far from the hospital.

I found a spot close to the building. Kathy and I locked the car doors and headed to the main entrance. As we approached the building, an ambulance pulled toward the far side of the hospital. There wasn't a siren, so we knew it was a DOA, short for dead on arrival.

The cafeteria was crowded, as usual. We made our selections then headed for a table in the back. We ate our breakfast and wondered which of the people in the cafeteria were part of The Group. What about that group at the end table? Maybe the people huddled and whispering at the front table were in on it, too. Would we ever know?

"Look, Jenny, there goes Chloe, and she's in a big hurry. She's running to the elevator. It's another half hour before we have to be on the floor. What do you suppose is happening?"

I quickly took the last sip of my coffee and picked up my tray to clear the table.

"Let's go follow her. We'll pretend that we wanted to check the board ahead of time to see where we're assigned today."

We disposed of our trash and headed toward the elevator. As we entered, we heard two nurses discussing another murder. The victim was a nurse who transferred to the records department several years ago.

"What happened to her?" I asked. My curiosity got the best of me. "Oh, I'm sorry. My name is Jenny, and this is my friend, Kathy. We work in the O.R. We just came on duty a few seconds ago. I couldn't help overhearing your conversation and was wondering who you were talking about, and how she was murdered."

The older nurse eyed the younger nurse, but I guess she figured it was public knowledge at this point.

"Well, in the paper this morning it said that the Sheriff received a call from one of the woman's daughters. Seems she hadn't heard from her mom who normally called every morning. When the mom didn't call, the girl became very concerned and called the Sheriff's office. When they went out to her house, the Sheriff found her with a plastic bag over her head and there was a note attached. Someone said the most recent newscast reported that the note said something about her being too nosy, but I don't know. Like I said, she worked here in the records department," the younger nurse explained.

She looked to the older nurse who nodded, and then she leaned in closer to me to whisper, as if there was anyone other than us in the elevator.

"I think she was looking into something about the organ cases. She was questioning reports regarding the donors. Rumors are circulating that papers were not being filled out and that some of them had been forged." She returned to her previous stance and volume. "I don't know. It's scary though."

Her friend nodded in agreement. The elevator doors opened to our destination.

"Yes, very scary. Thanks for the info. Nice to meet you both," I said.

Kathy and I stepped out of the elevator. I looked back and the nurses waved as the doors closed behind me.

"Jenny, did you know her? I mean the lady who was murdered?" Kathy whispered.

"No, not really. I have seen her around here and there, in the cafeteria a few times, and we would make small talk. She would call up to the O.R. from time to time asking for records. She hasn't called me lately, though which is kind of strange. But, no, I didn't really know her."

Our spirits were quickly sinking. We were in danger. Neither one of us knew what to do nor how to help ourselves or anyone else involved. We couldn't trust a soul and we certainly couldn't talk to anyone about this. We were hoping to spot Chloe to see what she was up to, but she was nowhere to be found.

We changed into our scrubs in the nurses' lounge then walked to the main area outside the operating rooms. No one was there. The room where the extra supplies were held, normally busy with people going in and out, was also empty. The lights were on in the room we were caught peeking into yesterday. I looked at Kathy, and she looked at me. We decided to play it safe for now and not go anywhere near that room. Instead, we checked the nurses' schedule for the day. We were shocked to see that Chloe was scheduled in the closed-up operating room. This was a dead giveaway; Chloe knew everything. We were now certain of her involvement.

Kathy and I stared at the closed operating room. Since Chloe was in on the organ transactions, it was also possible that she was involved in the patients' deaths, too. She was just as dangerous to us as the others in the Code Blue Search Group. To unravel this mystery would take a modern-day miracle. We were both quietly thinking when we heard a door slam behind us. Kathy and I both jumped as if we'd been shot from a cannon. Twirling around, we looked into the eyes of Dr. Kenalog.

"Well now, young ladies. You are both on time this morning. The case will start in fifteen minutes."

"Yes, sir, Dr. Kenalog. We were just trying to find Chloe, actually. She got on the elevator, and appeared to be in an awfully big hurry. We were wondering if something was wrong with her or her dad. Is everything okay?" I asked trying to sound genuinely concerned.

"I'm sure she is perfectly capable of attending to herself," Dr. Kenalog replied.

"We were just wondering. I guess we'll try to catch her later." I shrugged.

With a look of disgust, he turned and walked away.

"Jenny, why did you act like we were concerned about Chloe? We know where she is. What's wrong with you?"

"Kathy, do you not recall our recent discussion about playing dumb? And I mean real dumb."

Kathy and I were assigned to O.R. number three with Dr. Kenalog. When we walked into the operating room, we saw the draped body. It was in the prone position with the head facing the door. The back table was set up. There were two masked faces standing at the table. A new face neither one of us recognized was also present. We took our places beside the body. Kathy and I both gasped when we looked at the dead body's face. It was the nurse who had worked in the records room; the nurse who was murdered. Dr. Kenalog walked in and strolled to the head of the table.

"Okay, team, this is an unusual case. The reason is that it is a murder case. The patient was dead when we got the call, obviously, but we don't know the exact time of death. We pronounced her deceased when the team arrived. She's being infused with certain fluids that will prevent discoloration. We will perform a special procedure on her, and that is why some of you have been handpicked, if you will. You will be participating in a new procedure today. It hasn't been performed in this little town before, but it has been done many times in larger towns around the world."

Kathy and I glanced at each other. Neither one of us dared to breathe a word. The others said nothing. I noticed nothing appeared to be wrong with the body. There were no marks, discoloration, or anything. It was like the body I had seen in the closed off room. Unknown fluid was running through the IV.

"Okay, ladies and gentlemen, let's begin the new procedure," said Dr. Kenalog.

No one but Kathy and I seemed to be frightened. The rest of the medical team just stood there looking unconcerned. I sensed this was not the first time for this so-called new procedure.

"Okay. We will now turn the head and place it in the table opening for better accessibility. Now, please observe as I bore a small hole in the base of the skull; it will be the size of a half dollar, or maybe slightly bigger. You will get the reasoning behind it when you see the outcome. During each step of this procedure, please pay close attention as I explain what I am doing." He started drilling as we observed.

The others gave no evidence of being interested in the so-called new procedure. After making the hole, Dr. Kenalog held out his hand and said, "The object, please."

The tech picked up what appeared to be a case that held a metal, or perhaps steel, object from the mayo table beside him. Dr. Kenalog took the object out of its case and carefully checked it. There were tiny wires running in and out of the device. It was something reminiscent of the Twilight Zone.

We continued to observe as he carefully inserted the object into the site of the opening. It was the exact size of the hole that he just drilled. Somehow, I knew from the way he handled himself and this procedure that he had done this many times before.

After the insertion was complete, Dr. Kenalog promptly commanded Kathy and me to leave the O.R. He stated the procedure was complete except for the final closure. No one else was asked to leave. Not a single one of them seemed to have any concerns about what just happened. I took mental notes about their attitudes and their actions. They never even asked a question. The teaching appeared to have been directed toward Kathy and me.

When we walked out of the O.R., we saw that the other operating room, the closed one, was still lit up.

"Go back and hide as close to the door as you can, Kathy, without being seen. Make sure that Dr. Kenalog is still busy, and that no one comes out without alerting me. Don't let me get caught again whatever you do."

"Okay, but hurry, because if you're caught, then so am I. Please Jenny, just hurry,"she begged.

I walked to the door and eased it open quietly. I looked in and saw a patient hooked to an IV. The position was the same as in the case we just completed. Chloe was at the head of the table and was actually doing the same procedure that Dr. Kenalog had just done. She had her back to the door, and the others were standing there doing nothing. There was no back table set up. I turned and saw Kathy still waiting and watching. I eased back over, got her by the arm, and we headed to the lounge to change.

"What did you see in there?" Kathy asked.

"The same procedure that we just did with Dr. Kenalog, but guess who was doing it this time?"

I slipped into my casual clothes waiting for Kathy to make the correct conclusion.

"Who? Dr. Evans?"

C'mon Kathy, think! I bit my tongue.

"No, not Dr. Evans. Actually, it was little Miss Chloe. And she was doing it all by herself."

I made a sweet, innocent face for effect; then turned to the mirror to take off my nursing hat and fix my hair.

"She what?" Kathy finally gave me her undivided attention.

"Yes, she had the drill and was doing the same procedure. The others were just standing around looking unconcerned and talking, but I couldn't hear what they were saying. She was at ease doing that procedure. It was as if she had performed it so often that she could execute it in her sleep." I assumed this with a "*See, I told you so*" attitude.

"Let's get out of here now," Kathy said. She quickly zipped her skirt and put on her shoes.

We rushed to the parking lot. Our routine was to look all around the car in an attempt to make sure no bad guys were hiding in the back seat.

"We're going to call the Sheriff as soon as we get home." I made up my mind and that was that.

"I thought we learned that he is in on it," Kathy said like she remembered a detail that I did not.

Duh Kathy! As if I'd forget something so crucial! I swear sometimes this is like dealing with a child. Calm down, I tried to tell myself, *she's just trying to be helpful.*

"Not Sheriff Watson, Kathy! We are going to call the sheriff of Riverside County. It's a big town, and he is a really nice man. He used to go fishing with my dad during the summer. He's known our family since I was a kid; so tonight I'll call Dad to get his number. We'll start the ball rolling once and for all. I think it's time we act before time runs out!"

CHAPTER THIRTEEN

We pulled into the parking space at the apartment. Things looked quiet for the most part. There were a couple of teenagers hanging out on the corner. They were smoking and playing their boom box, but they didn't even look over in our direction. The afternoon was draped in sunlight and tranquility. The sky was beautiful. Everything seemed okay in the apartment, and we were glad. We were stressed and tired. This whole thing with the so-called Code Blue Search Group was taking its toll on both of us. Just as we sat down, the phone rang. We both jumped.

"Hello?" I answered.

"Jenny?" the male voice asked.

"Yes," I replied. *What now?* I was getting tired of these varied strange men who kept calling me.

"This is Dr. Evans. I called to inform you that there is going to be an urgent meeting at the hospital tonight. It is a mandatory thing, and I expect you and Kathy to be back here in two hours."

"Okay, but..." I tried to come up with a good excuse as to why we couldn't make it, but I had trouble with lying on the spot.

"See you then." Dr. Evans finished the one-sided conversation and hung up.

I placed the phone on the cradle and told Kathy what he said. There was nothing to do but be pulled back and forth in their game until we could get some help. It was 4:00 p.m.; we needed to be there at 6:00 p.m. We both decided that calling my dad to tell him what was going on would be a good thing to do before we left for the meeting. Kathy was an only child. She had lost her parents in a plane crash years ago. There wasn't anyone to worry about her.

As I dialed the number, I knew Daddy was going to ask a lot of questions, but I would have to give him the details later. Maybe the meeting would give me more information that would help the sheriff in Riverside County. Kathy and I could go to Dad and Mom's place on the weekend and tell them everything. The answering machine took the call.

"Dad, this is Jenny. I just wanted to get some information from you. I want to call the sheriff there and talk with him about some things, but I don't have the number. Please call me when you and Mom get in. I am getting along great, so don't worry about me. Okay, know that I love you both."

Before ending the call, it occurred to me that it had been a few weeks since I'd talked to either of my parents, which was out of the ordinary. Normally, we spoke every other weekend.

I'd become so involved in the puzzle overshadowing the hospital that I hadn't thought about the lapse in our communication.

"By the way, where have you two been the past few weeks? Call me back. Bye."

I hung up with a slight feeling of uneasiness but couldn't put my finger on it. Maybe they went to the cabin for a long weekend. They had a big garden and bought a few cows, chickens, and a couple of hogs. It had become their getaway, and it brought them a lot of happiness in their declining years.

"Let's try to get some rest before we have to leave," I suggested to Kathy. "Hopefully my parents will call back before then."

I decided to lie down on the couch. Sleep came, but not without taking me on a fitful journey to the unknown. Dreams took over and placed me in a narrow tunnel without an end. I could see a light, but every step I took toward the light took me deeper into the tunnel and darkness.

"Jenny, get up! We have to get ready to go." Kathy woke me with a poke.

Maybe a nap wasn't such a good idea. I felt more exhausted than ever. I straightened my hair, grabbed my purse, and headed to the door. Kathy was already out in the car. We headed to the hospital. I was still wondering why Dad and Mom hadn't called, but I would definitely drive there this weekend. It was time for me to see what was going on with them.

We pulled into the hospital parking lot, which was jam-packed with cars. Most of the vehicles appeared to be from out of town. We had to drive to the next block to find a parking place. We caught the shuttle bus and rode to the hospital. The driver appeared dazed and said nothing to us. He was a strange man all dressed in black clothes and he wore a black hat that was pulled down low on his head.

"How long have you worked here, sir?" I asked trying to gauge whether he knew what was going on.

The man looked up and examined me in the rear-view mirror, but he didn't answer. *Maybe he didn't hear me.* I hoped that was all it was.

We got out at the front entrance of the hospital. The driver pulled away and headed to the back lot. We stared at the shuttle as we walked to the front door.

"What floor is the meeting on, Jenny? Do we have a clue?"

"No, we'll just go to the nurses' lounge, find Chloe or one of the doctors, and ask."

We got on the elevator. Dr. Evans stepped out of nowhere and got on with us.

"Hi, ladies, I am glad that you made it on time. It is indeed a big night for all of us. It's like a coming out meeting, you might say. Have you heard of coming out balls or cotillions? Well, this is along the same lines.

A number of people and other things of interest are to be introduced to you tonight."

He grinned like the cat that ate the canary. It was very unsettling.

"Yes, sir, I'm sure it must be an important meeting to have us come back to the hospital so quickly." Kathy almost sounded enthused, but it didn't work.

"Where is Chloe, doctor?" I asked.

"She is in the meeting room with the other visitors." He smiled again.

"Oh, and where is the meeting, sir?" Kathy asked.

"On the sixth floor, of course." He pointed to the lit number on the elevator panel. "That's a very private floor used for special events."

"The sixth floor? No one goes to the sixth floor." Kathy's words fumbled out of her mouth. "I mean the elevator keys are always blocked and we have never even…"

The elevator stopped with a jolt. Dr. Evans seemed to be smiling within himself. I never even noticed that he inserted a key into the panel before pressing the "6" button. Kathy was right; usually access to this floor was strictly prohibited.

"Okay, ladies, we're here."

Dr. Evans held the door open, removed his key, and motioned for us to walk ahead of him. We stepped out of the elevator and found ourselves surrounded by crosses, strange paintings of black dogs, daggers, and other sinister-looking objects. The eeriness of the décor was indescribable.

"Wait here, ladies, and I will be back to get you in a few moments." Dr. Evans was practically frothing at the mouth with anticipation.

What the hell is going on? I wondered as I began to tremble and my stomach churned. I felt that our end was just beginning; there would be no ending at all. This place reminded me of a television show that I once watched about satanic rituals. *Would we be tortured and killed by these sickos?* There was no way out. The elevator doors closed and there were no buttons on this floor to open the door back up, just a keyhole.

Kathy and I huddled together on a nearby red sofa—too afraid to move. The carpet underneath our feet was a dark color, almost black. There were pictures of wizards and crosses hung along the length of the long hallway ahead of us. The doctor went into a room at the far end of the hall. I looked at Kathy, and her face mirrored the terror I'm sure was displayed on mine. I examined the books that were piled next to us on the hall table. The titles were things about which I knew nothing. There was a book called the Al–Jilwah. There was a book about materials for doing various rituals, including something called Baphomet jewelry. There were also books on chanting and energy sources. All of it was Greek to Kathy and me.

"Did you know this place was here?" Kathy's voice had an uncontrollable tremor to it.

"No, I didn't. No one was ever allowed to come up here. The elevator was always on lock, and I thought it was a place where hospital property and such was stored. You know, just important things. But, I think…Shhh, somebody's coming."

Kathy gripped my hand so tightly that it was beginning to go numb. The elevator opened and several men in black hats and suits stepped off. They were walking in unison, carrying black briefcases. We watched as they filed past us, never batting an eye or looking in our direction. They walked down to the room that Dr. Evans had gone into. The light that emitted from the open door of that room was dim. Suddenly, out stepped Dr. Kenalog and Dr. Evans. They came toward us. We were both holding our breath. It was time, and I felt in my spirit that things would never be the same.

"Okay, ladies, it's time for the meeting of all meetings; you'll be just as surprised as everyone that attends these meetings. I always look forward to them," Dr. Evans said. He smiled yet again while Dr. Kenalog hovered over us.

Kathy and I held onto each other's hand. We stood up from the couch and followed the doctors down the hall. We walked past all of the horrible pictures of dogs with the heads of people and other monstrous drawings. It felt like one of the longest walks I had ever taken. Dr. Kenalog led us into the room, and we saw why the lights were so dim. There were black candles burning all around the perimeter; the flames seemed to leap out in a faint blue glow as if beckoning with fingertips to each person in the darkened room. The place was huge and there were people seated in rows as far back as we could see. Their chairs were draped in black. The people turned and looked as we entered. They each had on strange looking headdresses with numbers written across the front. Upon entering, we were quickly ushered to the front of the room where we would be seated. The seating arrangement had been set up so that Kathy and I would be facing the group. Dr. Kenalog made his way up to the platform and began to speak. We sat there frozen.

"Ladies and gentlemen, I would like to welcome the newcomers along with some of our board members who were able to attend tonight. Many were not able to attend for reasons that are tied to our base project and their involvement in this mammoth endeavor. We are here tonight to discuss the greatest findings in all of medical history. You will actually have the opportunity to witness the beginning of this technology and what we have been able to do with it thus far."

Dr. Evans stepped up and whispered something in Dr. Kenalog's ear. Dr. Kenalog nodded and continued his speech.

"Since the beginning of mankind, we have worked with scientists and others in the field in order to come up with various ways to test things for the betterment of the world as a whole. At this time, I will start by introducing you to a group of people. Dr. Evans, would you bring them in, please?"

Dr. Evans stepped to a door in the back of the room and pushed a button. He spoke in a foreign language that was not familiar to me. A group of men and women filed in wearing black robes; they all wore scarves on their heads. We watched as they made their way to the front of the room, close to where Kathy and I were seated.

"Ladies and gentlemen, please remove your scarves at this time," Dr. Evans instructed.

They removed their scarves revealing heads without hair; some individuals had scars in the medial section of their foreheads, and other scars were located at the base of their skulls. We saw the nurse that had supposedly been murdered. Dr. Evans controlled their every move with a remote control. They all had the little minute chips that we had seen that day, implanted in their heads. I felt a hand on my shoulder, and I screamed as I looked around at the ghostly familiar man behind me.

"Hello, Jenny, dear. It's so good to see you. Mom and I are so glad that you and Kathy could join us. This is such a marvelous group, and we're growing so fast. You'll be so happy girls; so happy indeed. Why, they have big plans for you two, or so we've been told!"

I slid to the floor in this darkened room where the candles seemed to dance with another spirit. There were cobwebs surrounding me. Nothing mattered now. Hands carried me to the chasm from which there was no escape.

I drifted down into a hole of pitch black with one barely audible word escaping from my lips. "Daddy?"

CHAPTER FOURTEEN

I vaguely remembered drifting into what felt like a dark hole. Memories of the room with its black candles, dancing blue flames, and evil manifestations danced like puppets in my mind. The images were so vivid that only death could erase them from me.

Evil flashed in the darkened meeting room that night along with people who were floating in and out of the shadows with scarves on their heads. Laser beams appeared to be shining from their necks and heads where the microchips had been implanted. I couldn't begin to figure out what any of it had to do with the selling of human organs. I wondered just who Dr. Evans and Dr. Kenalog really were. Maybe I should have been concerned with what they were more than who they were.

My parents were now among the non-living. A part of me had died when I saw them. My own father and mother were no longer as I knew them. *How could this be happening?* I hoped I was dreaming and would wake up at any time.

Kathy and I were brought back to my apartment, but I couldn't remember how we had gotten there. I was in my bed. I didn't hear Kathy moving around, so I assumed she was asleep. I carefully climbed out of bed and my head began to spin like a top. I grabbed the dresser to keep from falling. Things were out of focus. A picture of last night pranced boldly before my eyes. My parents had entered into the room where the black candles were burning. Mom's head was covered with a scarf, and Dad had something around his neck. Now that I think about it, every one of them looked like robots or mannequins.

I held onto the dresser as I made my way to the bathroom. I splashed cold water on my face to clear the cobwebs from my head. I needed to make some decisions, and I needed to make them quickly. Kathy and I had to get out of town. Kathy was weak, and I wasn't feeling so bionic myself. I realized a long time ago that she was the weaker of the two of us. I would have to make all of the decisions and determine the best strategy from here on out.

I heard a knock on the front door. I managed to get my robe on while running and half falling to the entranceway.

"Who is it?" I barely squeaked out. My throat was so dry.

"Johnson, ma'am; I'm from the repair shop," the person on the other side of the door answered.

"I didn't call for a repair person. What address are you looking for?" *Oh please just go away*, I thought to myself.

"Is your name Jenny Warren?" he asked. Though I couldn't see him, I could tell by his voice that he was annoyed.

"Well, yes, but I didn't call for a repair man. Who sent you?" I was in no condition for visitors.

"Look lady, I ain't got all day long to hang out talking to no high falooten ol' door hole while you stand in there yelling out at me. I was sent by this guy, and I was told to do a job here. And now, I'm gonna call and tell 'em you wouldn't let me in to do my work. Are you gonna let me in there or not?"

He was angered, but I wasn't going to budge, not after all that we had just been through.

"No, Mr. Johnson. I'm not. I didn't call you; therefore, you will not be getting in to repair anything in this place. Go and call anybody you wish, but get away from here and do it pronto." I crossed my arms and leaned my back against the door. I could be tough when I had to be.

"Fine! Good day, ma'am!"

I peeked through the key hole. I could see the truck parked outside by the curb. It looked legitimate enough, but the name was not one I recognized, K-E-R, Inc. There had been no calls placed from here, so a red flag surfaced in my mind. I didn't think it could've been a simple misunderstanding. After all, he knew my name, and his timing was just too perfect.

Fear had become a constant companion. I was afraid at the hospital, of The Group, of receiving more phone calls; and most of all, I was afraid that more people would be dying. As I turned away from the door, I retrieved the photo of my parents from the mantle. I hugged it tightly and crumpled into a sobbing heap on the living room floor.

When I had no more tears left to cry, I knew I needed to shake off my grief and do everything in my power to bring these people down! I wanted to know about the chips: What did they do? Who controlled them? What programs were in them? Who implanted them in my parents? *How dare they bring my parents into this!*

The more I thought about it, the more my blood began to boil. Kathy was still asleep. I needed to get her up. We had to figure out how to get help for the remainder of the town. I walked into the hallway and knocked loudly on Kathy's door. I heard her moan. Maybe she was sick and not asleep after all. I felt sick too, when I first opened my eyes this morning. I knocked again, only louder. Kathy let out a piercing scream.

I swung open the door. I was relieved that she was alone.

"Kathy, it's me Jenny. Wake up. Stop screaming. You're having a nightmare. Kathy! C'mon wake up. Can you hear me? Wake up!"

I grabbed her shoulders and began shaking her. She opened her eyes and looked at me with a terror that penetrated my own spirit and she screamed even louder. I slapped her hard across the face, but she wouldn't stop screaming. I ran to the kitchen and grabbed the water pitcher. I ran back into the room. Kathy was sitting up in the bed with her eyes closed again, still screaming. I threw half the pitcher of ice water on her. Her eyes dropped open, her pupils were as big as saucers, but her screaming was finally silenced. I sat down beside her on the bed.

I wrapped my arms around her neck and instinctively rocked back and forth.

"Shhhhh Kathy, listen to me, okay? Things are going to be alright. Do you hear me? Everything is going to be fine. Do you understand me? You must listen to me." I released her, but held onto her chin and looked into her eyes to make sure she was cognizant. I wiped her hair away from her face and handed her a tissue. "Let's go get you dried off. Here, put on your slippers, and let's go into the kitchen. It was a dream, that's all. You have to try and put things into proper perspective, Kathy. We both must remain calm. Here, put on your robe before you get cold." I helped her into her robe.

She stopped me before walking out of the bedroom. She was terribly upset.

"It was a horrible nightmare, Jenny. There were dead bodies, and they were pulling on me. I screamed and turned around to look for you. I caught a glimpse of you in the corner at the far end of a long corridor and called your name. Your mouth was wide open, I turned to see what you were staring at and I saw your dad and mom. It looked like you were trying to scream at them, but the words would not come out. I don't know. They were laughing loudly and acting like they didn't know you. Jenny, tell me this isn't really happening to us. Tell me it's a hallucination or something, but please tell me it isn't real."

My poor dear friend was at the end of her rope.

"I wish I could tell you that, Kathy, but I can't. C'mon let's go out in the kitchen. I'll make coffee, and maybe we can sit down and come up with a plan."

It was dismal outside, like a storm was brewing. The wind howled, giving me the creeps. Any other time I may have enjoyed the moods of Mother Nature, but not on that day. Thankfully, we weren't scheduled to work; not that I was ever going back to that place, scheduled or not.

"Pour the coffee. I'm going to take the phone off the hook," I said.

Kathy's response startled me.

"Why are you taking the phone off the hook?"

"Because, I don't want to talk to anyone today, except for you. Half of the town is probably wearing those implants." I shook my head because it was all still so difficult to believe.

"Oh, Jenny, do you really think it's *half* the town?" Kathy doubted.

"Yes, Kathy, I do. I think it's at least half, and probably more. If we don't make some plans and follow through quickly, we won't have a chance in hell of getting out of here."

I continued into the living room with the intention of unplugging the phone jack altogether.

Out of the corner of my eye, I caught a glimpse of a shadow outside the garage door. There was no deadbolt lock on the laundry room door that led to the garage entrance. As a single female living alone, I thought it would be best to put deadbolts on all the doors when I moved in, but I never got around to putting one in the laundry room.

"Kathy, go to the other door quickly and lock the deadbolt." I motioned to her as I made a bee line to the front door.

"What for?"

"Ugh, just do it, Kathy!" I snapped.

She did as I ordered while I quickly locked the doorknob on the laundry room door. I also slid the dryer in front of it as much as I could. It wasn't enough to prevent a break-in, but at least it would buy us some time, if necessary.

"What happened?" Kathy stood in the doorway watching me like I was crazy.

"Someone is outside by the garage door. I just saw a shadow when I went in to take the phone off the hook. Pull the blinds and close the curtains. I don't want him to see that we're home."

Kathy got on all fours and crawled over to the window to pull the curtains closed. If anyone saw what we were doing, they would think that we were acting completely ridiculously.

"Let's call the police," Kathy suggested.

"No, we can't do that. What if we get Sheriff Morgan or one of his buddies on the phone? What if we get someone with a chip? No, just help me secure everything."

"And I suppose you think that we are going to sit here, and discuss what we need to do next as if nothing is happening? I mean, we don't know who is outside watching us. Do you remember when those men were sitting in the living room? They actually broke into your apartment. My God, what if they crawl down through the window up in the old attic or something?" Kathy looked up at the ceiling.

"They can't get in the attic door." I dismissed her theory. "That was sealed shut before I moved in here. Someone put locks on the outside, and it's well secured. Besides, we would be able to hear someone banging around up there. That room is the least of our worries."

Speaking of worries, I was mad at myself for not getting a gun permit sooner. We purchased the guns when we went to the store, but didn't realize we had to wait to be cleared for our permits before we could leave the store with them in our possession. The dealer told us that he had a shooting class starting the following week. He said by then we'd be able to get our permits, pick up our guns (which they held in the store safe for us in the meantime), and learn to shoot, all on the same day. With everything that was going on, it slipped both our minds. So now, we didn't have any protection.

Getting away from here was going to be all the more difficult.

"Okay. Let's draw on our intellectual side and work this out together. We must come up with a plan. The way things are going now, we must act in a hurry because we are running out of time. First off, Kathy, you have got to start being more cautious. We can't make irrational decisions."

"What did I do that was so irrational?" Kathy asked defensively.

"Well, for starters, who were you going to call when I told you there was someone outside by the garage?"

"The police. Isn't that what you're supposed to do? Is that not what most people do?" Kathy folded her arms like a stubborn child.

"Yes. Yes, indeed that's what anyone else would do. But, do they do it in a town where the police are in on all of the criminal activity? Where body parts are on sale to people in other places? Oh, and by all means, Kathy, let's call the same people who were at the coming out meeting doing a microchip fashion show!"

"Alright, alright, I see the picture you're painting. So I am dense in some areas. I'm not familiar with how to act in a town full of murderers. Is that what you are insinuating?"

"Look, Kathy, I know you're scared. I am, too. If we make one wrong choice, it can cost us everything, which right now means our lives. I think the first thing we need to do is get our finances in order. The income from our extra work should total up to a nice sum. I haven't touched any of the money in my account. Have you?"

I went over to the pile of mail that I had been neglecting. I ripped open my most recent bank statement to verify how much was in there.

"No, I haven't. I was going to buy a new car a few weeks back, but for some reason I never got back across town to the car dealer; so I really should have a tidy sum in my account too."

"Okay, the apartment is paid up for several months, so we should be okay."

I sat on the couch with my pile and continued opening up my mail. The bills would need to be paid if we were going to leave town for awhile. I didn't want my credit rating to be ruined in addition to everything else that was being destroyed in my life!

"You know, Jenny, I remember you saying that you weren't going to run from anyone or anything. I can't believe you're talking about doing this."

Kathy sat down opposite me and grabbed my hand. I pulled my hand out from her grasp and stood up to explain myself.

"Kathy, when I said that, it appeared that a few people were involved in the sale of human organs. Now, I am sure that it extends far deeper and is more deviant than I realized. After seeing those chips being implanted and knowing that they are altering the victims, I think we are in an underground operation of some major proportions. We must get out of here. Our lives depend on how we handle things. The worst part of all this is that we don't know who our enemies are, where they are, or how widespread this thing is. From now on, we're going to have to think about everything before we act. Everything we do can have severe consequences. It could be days, months, even years before we can relax, if ever."

Kathy stood up and began to pace.

"Oh, please, Jenny. Why don't you just lock me in a room somewhere or go without me? I don't seem to be able to think properly anymore. I can't deal with this. Daddy and Mama used to tell me that I was such a smart child, but that I didn't have one smidgen of common sense to go with it. It seems that all I've done in the past few days is apologize for my poor decisions. Where would we go if we did leave, and what about your parents? I can't see how you can leave them. What are you going to do about them?"

The question jabbed into me like a dull knife. I swallowed back my tears and forced out what I'd been feeling.

"I don't consider them as being my parents any longer. I just can't."

Kathy gasped at this revelation.

"How can I call them my parents? They're being controlled by electrical gadgets.

As far as I'm concerned, they're merely puppets."

I broke down at the thought of seeing them in that way. I wondered if I'd feel worse if they had been killed. I just wasn't sure. If I had to guess, I think my feelings of grief over their deaths would be pretty similar to what I was feeling now. The loss would be the same—I would never be with them again.

"I feel so badly now. I didn't mean to make you cry. I just thought that …well you know my parents were killed so long ago, and I miss them terribly. I thought maybe it would be hard for you to leave your mom and dad. I know they aren't the same, but at least they're still alive."

The dull knife stabbed me once again. I wiped away my tears and stepped back from Kathy who was patting me on the back in an effort to console me.

"Let's change the subject." I wiped my eyes again and dried the back of my hands on my pants. "I'll go get the maps and let's figure out where we are going. California is a big state. Maybe we could move to a real populated area like Los Angeles or San Francisco."

Kathy's mood lightened at the mention of a getaway.

"I was thinking the same thing! Since we are experienced nurses, we should be able to find jobs in a large city."

I pulled the atlas off the bookshelf. It contained fairly detailed maps of each of the 50 states. After glancing over the map of the U.S., Kathy's adventurous nature took over.

"I was also thinking about Utah. You know they have the big Mormon college there. What's the name of it? Brigham Young or something like that? But, I don't like the mountains in the winter because of all the snow. How about southern Utah?" she asked. Her eyes lit up with excitement.

"Yes, we could buy an apartment and settle down and live a normal life again," I replied, resisting the urge to give her a reality check.

As we flipped through the pages, we discussed the pros and cons that went with each destination. Eventually, we came up with a tentative plan that satisfied both of us.

"What do we do about going to work tomorrow?" Kathy asked.

"We do absolutely nothing," I replied. "We won't call in because we would be picked up for sure. They aren't going to let us out of The Group now. For the most part, we're ready. Why don't we just leave today?"

Kathy's child-like deviant grin lit up her face at first, but then, after thinking more about it, she frowned. We both knew it wasn't going to be an easy task.

"What about the phone? Should we leave it off the hook?

If they call and get a busy signal, don't you think that someone might come out here pretty soon to see what the problem is?" Kathy asked.

"You're right. Put the phone back on the hook. We'll leave on a small light so that it looks like we've gone out for the evening. Maybe leave on the porch light, too."

"Okay." Kathy followed my suggestions.

I headed into my bedroom as I was trying to think of all that I would need to pack. Within moments, Kathy was standing in my doorway.

"I put the phone back on the hook, but there wasn't a dial tone when I picked it back up to check it. What's up with that?"

Without looking up I answered, "I'm sure it takes a second, Kath. Just give it a few seconds." I waved her off, but she stayed in the doorway.

"Wait a minute. We can't leave yet," she said.

Is she trying to be irritating? I stopped packing to play her annoying little game.

"What are you talking about now? Why can't we leave yet? It's daylight outside."

"Sure it's daylight, but what about the guy you saw outside? He could still be out there waiting for us."

I shook my head trying to refocus on my task.

"I'm sure he would have made a move by now if he were going to try anything. Now why don't you go get your stuff packed up?"

She finally left me in peace. This was completely out of character for me. I was one of those people who was always prepared and on time. The word "spontaneity" didn't exist in my book. If I knew I was going on a trip, I would've been planning out what I was going to take a couple of weeks in advance. As the days got closer, I would've had all my clothes dry-cleaned, my outfits and coordinating shoes picked out, and even my snacks for the trip would have been selected and ready to go. Unfortunately, this trip wasn't planned and I felt far from prepared, but we needed to leave as soon as possible. *This is as good as it is going to get,* I thought to myself as I zipped up my suitcase and rolled it into the hallway.

I paused to look back at my bedroom. It wasn't much, but it was all mine. I had a place for every blanket, every pillow, every piece of clothing, and every piece of furniture. Some of it was bought and some of it was given to me as gifts or hand-me-downs from my parents. I thought how strange it was that some objects brought vivid memories to mind, while others were just things. I silently prayed that this wouldn't be the last time that I would walk out of my apartment. I knew most of it was just "stuff," but the sentiment that went with some of the pieces was irreplaceable, especially now. I sighed and closed the door behind me. Kathy was waiting for me at the front door.

"I'll hide behind the curtains and peep out. Turn off all of the lights except for the one in the living room and the light over the stove. Set your suitcase by the door next to mine," she said.

We were about to walk out the door when the phone rang. I stared at Kathy and she stared at me. The answering machine picked up the call. A gruff, male voice came over the speaker.

"Hello, this is Mr. Wayland from the service center. We received your call to disconnect your phone service but we can't get to your area until next week. Someone will call and reschedule before coming. If you need other assistance regarding this matter, please call and ask for Betty. Thank you."

"Kathy, did you call the phone company to turn off our service?"

"No, of course not. Why would I do such a thing?"

"Something's not right. We need to leave, now." I felt the need to take control of the situation immediately. "Let me look out the window. You grab the suitcases. When I say it's safe, you take as much as you can to the car. I'm sure that whoever was hanging out there is gone by now."

Kathy nodded. I looked out, gave her the thumbs up, and we were off.

"Let's go, Kathy, the coast is clear. I'm right behind you. "

CHAPTER FIFTEEN

We walked outside into the drizzling rain. It took a few seconds to load our belongings into the trunk. I looked around the neighborhood. The elderly couple across the street was under their carport. Both of them were on their hands and knees looking for something. They were always doing strange things over there.

"Okay, we'll head straight to Dover Bank then hit the interstate. We'll figure out where we're going from there." I numbered my mental checklist.

We pulled into the parking lot of the bank. It was very busy. People were coming and going in a hurry. I turned off the car and made sure that I had Kathy's full attention.

"Okay, we are going to walk in, fill out our paperwork, get our cash, and then we're out of here. We must look at the tellers closely so we can determine who we will approach. We should avoid any tellers who have their heads or necks covered like the people with the chips had at the coming out meeting."

Kathy nodded in agreement and we got out of the car on a mission. There was a guard standing at the door of the bank, but he was busy talking to a couple of other patrons. They didn't look at us as we walked through the door. The bank was full of activity. It would be easy for us to blend in, take care of our business, and get out of there without any problems.

"Let's go to the kiosk and take a look around. We can pick out our tellers," Kathy whispered.

"Look," I said, pointing to the tellers, "there are two girls side by side, and they both have high-neck blouses on, but the man next to them is dressed in a shirt unbuttoned about the neck. What do you think?"

"I think you would make a pretty damn good detective and need to get into another line of work. You have touched on a very important observation, Miss Detective. We don't want to go to them for sure," Kathy said.

"Excuse me, ladies, but aren't you two nurses at the local hospital?"

Both Kathy and I turned around and looked into the face of the man who had been on the operating table. I felt the blood drain from my face. I looked at Kathy, and she was as white as a ghost.

"Why, yes, we are. I remember you. Didn't you have a blood clot or something?" Kathy pretended that she wasn't sure of the details, but I knew she remembered him and every single detail of his case.

"You sure have a good memory, Ma'am." He was notably impressed with her. "Yes, a blood clot, or so that's what they told me; actually they were quite vague about the details. When they put me to sleep for the operation, apparently something went wrong. They had me awake within an hour or so and said whatever happened corrected itself.

They also said I was not a good candidate for the operation because they found out I had a bad infection somewhere. They said I needed some sort of medicine, so I could be cleared up before doing something. I don't know. It made no sense to me. They talked about a mechanism of some sort that I might have to get later. Sorry. To be honest, I feel like I have suffered a bit of amnesia. I'm supposed to go back in a few weeks and see some doctor by the name of Kena something. I'm sorry, I honestly don't recall..."

"Would it be Dr. Kenalog by chance?" Kathy asked.

"Yes, that's right. Dr. Kenalog. He seemed to be a nice fellow for the most part. Well, ladies, I gotta go now. I have to get home and feed the farm animals. Good to see you. Take care now."

He waved as he exited the bank. I grabbed Kathy's arm.

"Oh, Kathy. I was so scared. I am weak all over now. Just stand still for a few minutes and let my nerves get settled."

I could tell by the sudden bright-eyed look on Kathy's face that she saw something.

"Look Jenny, see the woman in the red blouse behind the window where the vault is?"

"Yes, what about her?" I looked around slowly to see who she was talking about.

"Her name is Linda. She's a part-time volunteer at the hospital. I've known her for a while. She is really nice. I didn't know she worked here, though. Let's go to her, or at least I will. She is dressed normally."

"Okay, Kathy, you go on over. Stay on your toes and keep your wits about you. I'll go to the older gentleman that's working next to her."

We split up and as I stood in line to speak to the man, I overheard the conversation at Kathy's window.

"Hey, Linda, remember me? I'm Kathy, from the hospital." Kathy smiled sweetly.

"No, I'm sorry, but I can't recall. Are you a volunteer like me?" the teller asked.

"No, but for the kind of pay we get for what we do, you could almost call it volunteering." Kathy's smile faded a bit. "Actually, I'm one of the nurses. I have been doing special cases for a while, but usually I am an operating room nurse."

Linda snapped her fingers as something Kathy said jogged her memory.

"Oh, now I remember you!" Linda smiled. "We've talked a few times about going on a cruise or taking a trip to Europe."

Kathy exhaled with relief.

"What can I do for you, Kathy?"

"I need to draw a large sum of my money out. I am purchasing a new car, and my friend and I are going to buy the apartment we've been renting.

We plan to do some remodeling, but we're taking a little vacation first," Kathy explained.

"Oh, that sounds fun. Are you going to Europe to see all of the sights, or is it business?"

Linda had the most animated look on her face. It actually made me giggle a little.

"No, just going to make it one of those 'get in the car and go where the mood strikes for that day' trips. You know? Haven't you ever wanted to do that?" Kathy replied.

"Oh, yes. I think that's exciting. If I weren't committed to the hospital for the next two months, I would love to go with you. Okay Kathy, I've pulled up your account. You have a balance of fifteen thousand, one-hundred and thirty-two dollars. Does that sound right to you?"

"Yes, I think that's about what it should be."

"Well let's see. When you draw out a large sum like this, I have to put down the reason for it. I will have to get the bank manager to sign it, but that shouldn't be a problem. Wait right here, and I'll be right back," Linda said.

"Great! And thanks for getting things taken care of so quickly," Kathy called out.

Meanwhile, the elderly teller called me up to his window. I was able to give pretty much the same speech as Kathy and the results were fairly similar.

The man appeared to be at ease with my request and he was smiling, so I figured there wouldn't be any issues.

Linda returned to talk to Kathy while my teller was getting my paperwork in order.

"Okay, Kathy, the manager is in an important meeting, so I talked to his secretary and told her your situation about the house and car purchases. She said she would sign the documents, and you can be on your way. Do you want it in small bills or large bills?"

"I believe both small and large bills, Linda, since I will be traveling. People don't always want you to hand them large bills."

"Okay. Let's get this counted out, and then you can get going. How exciting!" Linda squeaked with delight.

It sounded like Linda was genuinely thrilled at the thought of traveling, even if she wasn't the one going anywhere. I probably could have saved my teller the trouble of going through the same procedure as Linda, but I didn't want to bring any unnecessary attention to our large withdrawals. So when he came back to the window to explain that the manager was in a meeting, I nodded and pretended that this was news to me.

I saw Kathy headed for the door with an envelope. I could tell by the smile on her face that we were almost home free.

She turned and winked at me as she opened the door and left. I felt some relief.

"Okay ma'am, here you go. Is there anything else I can do to help you today?" he asked while handing over my money.

"No. Thank you so much. That will be all," I replied.

I headed to the door as quickly as possible. I saw Kathy sitting in the car. She was on her cell phone, but didn't look upset.

"Yes, I did call to inquire about a map. Okay. Yes, that would be fine," Kathy said into her phone.

"A map? From the triple A?" I mouthed as I got into the driver's seat.

Kathy nodded as she listened to the person on the other line.

"Good thinking," I whispered.

"Thank you. We're on our way now," Kathy said and ended her phone call.

Kathy squeezed my hand. She was practically bouncing out of her seat with joy.

"Oh, Jenny, I'm so glad to see you with your envelope. We did it! Did you have any problems?"

I shook my head and buckled up.

"Smooth sailing all the way. Mr. Sutton was tired; he said he had two more weeks until he retires and then he's heading to Arizona. He said something about a cabin in the mountains; fishing, hunting, and becoming a hermit. Sounded a bit like our plans," I replied with a smile. "Kathy, I'm going to back this car out of here, and we are out of this town forever, or at least a long, long time."

I put the car in reverse, but Kathy startled me as I eased off the brake.

"Oh, be careful!" Kathy pointed. "The guards are looking at something over here. They're probably not looking at us, but drive cautiously anyway. We don't need any problems now."

I looked in my rear-view mirror and felt a bit relieved by what I saw.

"Oh, look behind us, Kathy. There's a fender bender in the parking lot. *Phew!* I'll drive around behind the drive thru instead."

We drove along for a few moments in silence. We were stunned that our plan was actually falling into place.

"All right, Kathy, we're on our way," I piped up, stating the obvious. "We'll go to the AAA Motor Club, get our map, and be gone. I am so excited about this decision. We have our money, and we made it out of the bank without any issues. I am all for not talking about this nightmare for a few days. How about you?"

"I totally agree, Jenny! I'm excited, too. I haven't felt this happy in weeks. Let's celebrate!

We should stop for dinner at a fancy restaurant, order a bottle of zinfandel, hors d'oeuvres, and have lobster Newburg. Maybe we can find a good theatre. Go see a play and forget about everything."

I allowed Kathy to get carried away. It all sounded so wonderful, but the pessimist in me wanted to spoil the fun. Instead, I decided to let her ramble on and I just smiled. It felt good to be free. There was no harm in enjoying it while it lasted.

CHAPTER SIXTEEN

Kathy and I were almost out of California when the fog settled around us. It wasn't dark but would be soon. We were both hungry and decided to look for a restaurant. The fog was getting thicker, and visibility was becoming almost impossible. We were in a town called Needles. It was on the state line between Nevada and California. The famous Route 66 ran through the middle of the town.

"Hey Kath, I think since the fog is so thick we may have to stop for the night. It's another 138 miles from here to Las Vegas, and it's too foggy to attempt the drive."

Kathy looked up from her magazine and agreed with my suggestion.

"Sounds great to me, Jenny. I'm starving anyway. That looks like a nice place over there."

She pointed over to a restaurant as we sat at a red light. When the light changed, I slowed to look for a parking spot in front of it.

"The sign says formal attire only, Jenny. I don't want to drag those suitcases out and change clothes now. Do you?"

"No, not really," I replied. "Let's drive down the road a piece. Surely there must be something that's open and casual in a town this big. It's not too late."

"I can barely see anything. The lights look like blurs in the fog," Kathy said. "I see a light flashing just ahead. Maybe that's a place to eat."

But as we got closer, I realized it wasn't.

"Nope, I guess not. They must be working on the roads. It's just one of those warning lights."

"Look, Jenny." Kathy pointed up the road. "That looks like a truck stop up there, or something. Do you want to go in there?"

I was squinting to try to see what she was talking about.

"No, not really, but since I can't see well enough to drive right now, I suppose we better stop before I wreck the car and kill us both."

As I pulled up to the place and circled the parking lot, Kathy noted, "It doesn't look too bad. Look at the crowd of people in there. The food must be okay for there to be that sort of crowd."

I agreed the crowd looked decent from the outside. At this point, I was just happy to be out of the driver's seat. We went inside and the place was buzzing with people. Some were dressed in casual wear and others were in business attire. The food smelled delicious and was set up buffet style. We sat down at a table next to a group of elderly men. All of them must have been hard of hearing because they were talking loud enough for everyone in the place to hear them.

"Hey, ladies. My name is Ms. J. What can I get you to drink?" the well-fed waitress asked.

"Hi, Ms. J. Is that short for Joan, Janice, or Jennifer?" Kathy asked out of genuine curiosity.

"Nope. It ain't short for nothin'. Mama says J was good enough for her and easy ta spells. What can I get you girls to drink?"

Kathy hid behind her menu while Ms. J waited for our response. She had her pen and pad ready for our order.

"Well, I think I will have a large iced tea with light sugar and lemon."

I smiled up at Ms. J, but she was too busy jotting down my order to notice me.

"Now, let me see… since we're going to stay the night, I think I'll have a highball," Kathy said.

"Sorry, miss, ain't any highballs on the menu here. You's in a truck stop, ma'am, not a club or anything like that," Ms. J replied.

She stood there with pursed lips waiting on Kathy who was now fumbling the menu nervously around in her hands.

"Oh, I see. Well, uh, bring me a glass of lemonade then with a twist of lime, oh, and a cherry." Kathy smiled and sat back, obviously satisfied with her new request.

Ms. J sighed.

"Ain't got no cherries neither ma'am. The delivery guy didn't come today."

C'mon Kathy! Why do you have to be so complicated? I thought to myself.

"Okay. Just the lemonade then and don't worry about what you don't have. Okay, Ms. J?" Kathy replied sweetly.

"Yep. I reckon that's what I'll have to do, miss. Y'all can grab your plates at the bar over yonder and help yourselves to some fine country cooking." Ms. J pointed to the buffet with her chin and walked away to get our drink order.

"Come on, Kathy, dear. Just help yourself to some good country cookin'." I mimicked Ms. J and led the way to the bar, walking like I just got off a horse.

"Jenny, stop!" Kathy whispered. "She's going to hear you and see you making fun of her. She scares me! I'm afraid she'll tie us to some wagon and drag us out into the desert to die."

I laughed at Kathy's ridiculous imagination.

"Oh, Kathy, for Pete's sake, relax. I'm just kidding! Have a little fun, why don't you? Let's hustle up some grub, woman," I said using my best John Wayne accent.

Kathy was flustered.

"Stop talking like a hillbilly and act like a professional."

It was fun to watch her take on the parenting role because of my child-like behavior. Usually she was the one who was being embarrassing.

"Okay, okay, I'll settle down." I reassured her. "Once we finish eating, we'll need to find a place to sleep for the night. We can ask Ms. J. to give us directions to the closest decent hotel."

"Alright, Jenny, but just behave now. Okay?" Kathy was still in parenting mode.

"Okay, Kathy, okay," I replied.

We ate in silence as everyone around us talked loudly about their business and family matters. We were tired, and the stress was catching up with us.

"Okay, ladies, what else can I get for you tonight? Would you wanna cup of coffee or somethin'?" Ms. J asked.

"No, Ms. J., we'll pass." I wiped my mouth with my napkin and said, "However, we would like to know where we can find the closest hotel. It's so foggy out tonight. We'd rather wait till morning to continue with our trip."

"Hmm," Ms. J thought for a moment, and then continued, "there's a bed and breakfast on the next block on the right-hand side. There's a swing and signs in the front yard. It's a real classy place, I hear; so try that."

"Thank you, Ms. J," Kathy said.

Ms. J forced a grin as she cleared our plates. We paid our bill at the register.

On her way to place the tip on the table, Kathy called back to me.

"I'm going to run to the bathroom real fast, Jenny."

"Okay." I nodded. "I'll join you."

While Jenny entered the stall, I stood back waiting in line. *Geez, is there a place on Earth that doesn't have a line in the women's bathroom?* While I stood quietly, I couldn't help but hear the conversation between two of the stalls.

"What did they do with 'em, Martha?" the first voice asked.

"Don't nary a soul know. Just takes 'em and disappears with 'em, Clara. Lord Jesus of this world, please helps us, I pray. Please, Lord, come down and helps us afore things get beyond control here, now," another woman replied with a Southern accent.

One of the women flushed and exited her stall. She was a little bit of a thing. I knew it was rude to eavesdrop, but I heard what I heard. With everything that was going on, I figured it wouldn't hurt to ask about it, just in case.

"Excuse me, ma'am. I couldn't help but hear your conversation. Did someone steal your money or break in your homes?"

The little lady began washing her hands as her friend exited from her stall.

"Oh, nah, miss. We didn't mean to troubles you none, but someone is a stealing signs all around here, and we is members of the First Holy Church of Believers, and we just knows what is going on, that's all. We just knows, miss. We do. The Bible tells us plainly what that ol' devil is up to, and it ain't no good, miss. It just ain't," she replied.

She dried her hands and looked to her friend.

"Let's go, Clara. We needs to get home and get in and lock our doors."

Clara wiped her hands as well and took the other lady's arm. I think I heard Clara call the little lady Martha as they headed for the door.

Martha stopped Clara and turned back to me to say, "Goodnight, miss. Now you be careful out there. Lock your doors and don't open 'em for anyone. Do you hear me, now? Lawdy mercy, sweet Jesus, help us. Please help us."

She shook her head and shuffled a few more feet. I stopped them from leaving.

"But, ladies, please tell me what is being stolen of yours. I would really like to help you," I insisted.

"It ain't ours, miss. It's dem signs of the Devil. All signs of the times. Oh, Lawdy Jesus, have mercy on us. Yes, ma'am. That is exactly what it is you see. He has his masters out getting 'em. It's comin' on to that time now. We gotta go, Miss. Lawd Jesus knows they be the only ones that want dem signs with all dem 6s on 'em...better reads your Bibles, ma'am," Martha added.

She hobbled out the door with Clara leading the way. Kathy was washing her hands at the sink behind me.

"What was that all about?" she asked.

I couldn't get out of there quickly enough. I rushed out to the car and Kathy followed closely behind me. We got into the car and I stopped before turning the key.

"Something about what they were saying, or not saying, tied in with us or what just happened in Morganville. I just know it does."

"Jenny, to be honest, I could hardly understand what she was saying. Something about signs and 6's and reading your Bible...the stuff she was saying really freaks me out, but, how could that have anything to do with what's happening in Morganville? I hope she was just being overly dramatic."

"I pray that you're right," I replied. "Let's go find a room and go to bed. I'm so tired. I can't think anymore. I was just getting relaxed and now this."

We drove down the street and made it to the bed and breakfast despite the limited visibility. It would do for tonight. Tomorrow we would head out for the next town. Las Vegas here we come!

CHAPTER SEVENTEEN

A beam of light was shining through the mauve-colored curtains. The sun pried its way through the mesquite trees making colorful patterns on the bedroom wall.

As I looked around the room, I was happy that we had asked Ms. J. about a nearby place to stay for the night. The decor was a pleasing Southwestern style. I crept out of bed and looked across the room at the other bed. Kathy was sound asleep. I decided not to wake her.

There was a fresh pot of coffee in the dining area. I poured myself a cup then opened the sliding door and stepped out onto the porch. An Old Yeller look alike sat perched on the back steps. He was a rugged sort of dog that looked as if he had seen his better days. This was an informal, comforting place that might actually help Kathy and I relax a little.

It felt good to get away from the dreadful smell of death at the hospital. It was crisp and cool outside. The birds were in melodious harmony as if rehearsing for a sing-along. Desert wildflowers bloomed all over the backyard and I could see mountains in the distance.

I thought of my parents as I admired the breathtaking view. When I was younger, I used to take trips to Vegas with Daddy and Mama every year. We would go up to Mt. Charleston to stay a few nights in a cabin and ski in the early mornings. The trees would be full of powder-white snow. It looked like a winter wonderland. I remember Daddy holding my hand so tight when I stood close to the ledge as I looked down at the valley below. He was afraid my foot would slip and I would fall down onto the jagged rocks. The memories awakened my sadness about what had happened to my parents.

I looked at my watch and figured it was time to wake Kathy. It was going on 9:30. She had not slept very well. Neither of us did. She'd tossed and turned, keeping me awake until I finally crashed from pure exhaustion. I was really concerned about the women in the bathroom talking about the signs that had been stolen. *What would anyone do with those signs anyway?* I mumbled to myself.

I walked back to our room. Before I could wake Kathy, there was a loud knock at the door. *Who in the world could that be?* No one knew we were here. I peeked through the peephole and saw a stout, rosy-cheeked lady with a bonnet on her head. She looked like a nanny. I opened the door and she handed me the paper.

"I brought you the paper, dear. I'm sorry. I didn't mean to wake you," she said. Her smile was as warm as her big brown eyes.

"Oh, you didn't wake me, uh, Miss..."

"Spencer, honey, my name is Miss Spencer. Well, I should be going now. I have to assist with serving and clean-up this morning. Have a blessed day," she said.

I closed the door and turned around to see Kathy getting out of bed. She looked like she was sleepwalking.

"Wake up, sleepy head. You have to help me figure out what we are going to do."

I playfully bonked her on the head with the newspaper. She didn't appreciate it and swatted me away.

"Last night you were so wound up that you tossed and turned half the night. I thought for sure you were going to throw yourself right out of the bed onto the hard floor or, even funnier, maybe out into the flower beds or something. Wouldn't that be a sight to see? Florence Nightingale look alike found tiptoeing through the tulips," I joked.

"You know you are not as funny as you think you are, miss know-it-all. You should be worried too after hearing those women talking about God and the devil and signs being stolen from all over the United States. The more I think about it, the more it really gives me the creeps."

"Oh, Kathy, and the more I think about it, the more I think it was pure nonsense. I admit, at first I was a little frightened, but really, what could that stuff have to do with either one of us? Let's try to forget about it. Please, stop freaking out before you make yourself sick. You said it yourself, they were probably exaggerating anyway."

She wasn't convinced. I handed her the newspaper hoping to change the subject.

"Here, let's get some coffee and read the paper. We'll go out on the porch and relax.

There's not any real need for us to hurry, anyway. Are you hungry?" I asked.

"No, I'm not hungry. I'm just tired. And you're right, we have nowhere to be, we should just relax."

Grabbing my coffee, I headed out to the back porch with Kathy close behind. The breeze was cool, and it felt almost like autumn. Neither of us had received any calls from the hospital or The Group on our cell phones. We hoped they weren't looking for us, yet.

"What section of the paper do you want?" Kathy asked.

"Just give me anything except the sports page. I hate that page."

She handed me the comics, of course. I was somewhat engrossed in the day's funny section when my concentration was abruptly interrupted.

"Oh my god, Jen, listen. Here it is; as big as day in the paper. There's a long article all about it."

"What are you going on about?" I shot her an annoyed look over the top of the newspaper.

"The street signs," she rambled.

"Oh." My stomach did a flip. *Uh-oh, maybe she's right about this.* "What does it say?" I asked trying not to sound too alarmed.

"It says that signs have been stolen from several states. No one really knows why, but religious leaders have stated that the thefts have a biblical meaning. All of the stolen street signs have the number 666 on them. Many state officials believe the thieves are teenage pranksters."

Kathy put the paper on the table and started strumming her fingers as if to say, "Do you believe me now?"

"What does 666 mean?" I asked.

"How do I know?" She yanked the paper off the table. "There's a hole in the paper where the numbers are, and I can't read the rest of it."

She stuck her fingers through the hole to show me what she meant.

"Why are you so on edge about this? Look at how worked up you are again!"

"I don't know, Jenny. I can't put my finger on it. Something inside me keeps thinking something dreadful is going to happen to us, and it's going to be the biggest nightmare."

I had nothing to say. We continued reading the paper in silence. I knew the numbers 666 meant the workings of the devil or some sinister being, but I wasn't about to tell Kathy that! I shut my eyes and tried to close out the feeling of impending doom. Suddenly there was a loud knock at the door. I almost fell out of the chair. Kathy jumped up and hollered.

"Jenny!"

She caught me from falling over.

"Who's there...are you? Just a minute," she called out to the person at the door. "You fell asleep," she whispered to me. "We're on the deck at the bed and breakfast. Someone just knocked on the door. Should I get it?"

"I'll get it," I replied.

I jumped up and tripped over my feet on my way through the bedroom. I was still half asleep.

I opened the peephole and saw the cute little granny lady on the other side of the door. *What was her name again? Oh right, Miss Spencer!* I opened the door.

"Hi, again. Will you and your friend be checking out today, or shall we count you in for another night?" she asked. She tilted her head like a puppy who heard a strange sound.

"Uh, let me talk to my friend and see what she thinks. Won't you come in for a moment?"

I held the door open wider, gesturing for her to enter.

"Yes, yes, I will come in and wait."

Miss Spencer walked in and took a seat on the corner chair while I went out to speak with Kathy who remained on the deck. After a quick discussion, we decided to stay. We needed the rest and we were enjoying the relaxing atmosphere at this place.

"Miss Spencer, we have decided to stay another night. Could you please tell us what time we need to be dressed for dinner?"

She slowly rose from the chair. This was probably the first break she had all day. It was obvious that she was a hard worker. As a matter of fact, I was beginning to wonder if she was the *only* worker.

"Very well. Somewhere around 6:30 we'll put the food on the buffet table. You come and serve yourself, is that okay?"

I nodded. Then said, "Wait a minute, Miss Spencer. What should we wear?"

"It's casual, dear. Don't worry about dressing up." She smiled.

"Thank you, Miss Spencer. We'll see you then."

I almost felt like I should hug her or something. She just exuded a certain warmth about her. I couldn't help liking her even though I didn't even really know anything about her aside from her name.

The day passed by without much excitement. We enjoyed the peaceful setting. I couldn't remember the last time that I had nothing to do except read and watch TV. It was wonderful. For a moment, I actually forgot that we ran away from home.

"Jenny, I'm going to lie down for a little nap. I am totally worn out."

Kathy yawned as she slid under the covers.

"You know, I think I'm going to take a nap, too, Kathy. We'll go to dinner this evening and have a good time."

I walked over to my bed, slipped off my shoes, and put my head on the pillow. However, it was all of three minutes before Kathy was speaking again.

"Jen, before I take my nap, I just want to ask you if you saw that guy in the backyard this morning. He seemed to be watching us."

"What backyard? What are you talking about?"

I propped up on my elbows to look over at her.

"That brick house about three houses down the way. If you go out on the deck and look to the left, you'll see the house."

"Yeah, so what about the guy?" I asked.

"Well, he was walking close to the hedges when I saw him. His eyes met mine; then he quickly turned his head and pulled down the wide brim hat he was wearing. I think he has long, dark hair, and a mustache. I don't know. He just gave me the creeps."

Kathy fluffed her pillow.

"So, what's so peculiar about those things? Maybe he lives there and thought you were being a peeping Kathy. I see nothing unusual about what you've described. I swear, you're going to start imagining things next and the next thing you know, we will both have ulcers."

I plopped my head back down on my pillow. She could tell that I was annoyed.

"I guess you're right, Jenny. Just forget it. I suppose I'm just being way too suspicious. Can you wake me up in time to get ready for dinner?"

She turned her back to me.

"Yup, I'll set the clock so we won't oversleep. I don't have a clue what to wear, but I couldn't care less, myself."

I heard a dog barking somewhere in the distance. A church bell chimed ever so beautifully as it played for the city at large. I closed my eyes and wondered what would become of us in the days to follow.

CHAPTER EIGHTEEN

"Kathy, hey, wake up. It's 5:45 p.m. C'mon get up. Kathy, wake up."

"No! I'll shoot if you come any closer. I will kill you....both of you... please, stop. No!" Kathy yelled with her eyes closed.

"Kathy, wake up!"

I grabbed her shoulders and shook her hard. She was sobbing loudly. Once awakened enough to see me, she pulled me into a hug.

"Oh, Jenny, it was horrible. I can't tell you how ghastly that nightmare was."

"Kathy, it was only that, a nightmare. C'mon, get a grip on yourself. Dreams or nightmares are usually due to mind overload or something you've thought about a lot. You know that. It's not real."

"But you don't understand, Jenny. It was your parents. They were coming at me with scalpels, numbers, and something in a black bag. They had ugly smiles on their faces and said they had been picked out to induct us because you were their daughter. I had a gun and was about to shoot them. I was going to kill your parents. Oh, Jenny, may God forgive me for even dreaming such a horrific thing."

Kathy continued to sob. I held her shoulders and looked at her squarely in the face.

"Kathy, it was just a dream."

I pointed out the obvious, but then, a thought struck me. I stood up from the bed and began to pace.

"You know, I never really thought about my parents doing anything to me. But now, well, they aren't really my parents anymore. I guess they could try to do something to us because of me. My parents are the ones who could track me down better than anyone. They know that I have a birthmark on my right shoulder blade and a big scar on my left leg where I had surgery as a child. They know my habits and the things I would and wouldn't do. They have my birth certificate, my social security card, and other important papers in a lock box in their bedroom safe. I couldn't change my identity if I wanted to unless I lied on all of the paper work. I mean, yeah, I could change my hair color and clothes, but not my identification information," I rambled.

"Oh, Jenny, they wouldn't do something like that. I mean they wouldn't really come after us, would they?" Kathy asked nervously.

"Yes, Kathy, come to think of it, they *would* do such a thing because they are not controlled by human instincts, actions, or brain power any longer. They are machines now; controlled by people who are far more evil than I could have ever imagined. Yes…" I had trouble allowing the words to escape my lips. "My parents are what I'd consider our worst enemies."

Kathy gasped.

"I'm sorry, Jenny, I shouldn't have told you about the nightmare. Now you'll worry about something you never even dreamed of happening."

"No, you did the right thing, Kathy. Actually you did something of great importance, because now we know that we must be much more careful than I originally thought. They can trace us easily. We should be much more aware of our appearances—our hair color and how we dress, the things we do, the places we go, and such. All of those changes must be dealt with quickly. We mustn't make it so easy for them to find us. No, you absolutely did the right thing for both of us. Maybe in the long run you've saved our lives in some way."

I nodded as I formulated more plans in my head for our future. Unfortunately, we would have to live our lives on the run. This would take diligence, but our lives counted on it.

"Okay, let's just forget the nightmare and get on with the evening," Kathy said. "What are you going to wear tonight? I haven't the faintest clue of what I'm going to wear. Well, let's get ourselves dressed and maybe we'll meet someone interesting tonight."

Kathy flipped through her suitcase. I headed to the bathroom just as someone knocked loudly at the door.

"Who's at the door now?" Kathy's eyes bulged out of her head.

"I don't know," I whispered. "Just calm down. It's probably just the little cleaning lady again. Let's answer it together."

The knock grew louder. Slowly, we walked toward the door.

"Jenny, you look through the peephole, and I'll just stand beside you," Kathy said.

"Alright, but be quiet and don't move. Shh!" I carefully peeked out to see who was there.

"What do you see? Who's there?" Kathy whispered.

"It's a man with a wide brim hat on and dark glasses. He has a mustache and long hair. He's looking up and down the hallway."

Kathy almost jumped out of her skin.

"That's the man who was walking in the yard a few doors down! He had the mustache, and he was wearing a wide brim hat. I think he had long hair, but I really couldn't see it because of the hat. I told you he was staring at us! I told you, and you just thought I was being overly dramatic about the whole thing. Don't open the door Jenny, I beg you, please, please don't!"

Kathy clasped her hands in prayer position.

"Kathy, stop it now! Get yourself together. He hasn't done anything to justify your behavior. I am going to open the door."

Kathy took off and ran into the bathroom to hide.

"Gee, thanks for your support," I mumbled under my breath. I took a gulp of air and abruptly opened the door just enough so that my face fit in the gap. I hid the rest of my body behind the door. *Aren't I just the brave one?*

"Yes, can I help you, Mr.?" I asked.

"The name is Green, ma'am. Attorney Steven Green."

He held out his hand to shake, but I decided against reaching out. He pocketed his hand when he realized I wasn't reciprocating.

"Oh, uh, I'm supposed to tell you that dinner will be served early, and you ladies are invited to come down now." He paused and then added, "Uh, if you are dressed."

Did he actually think I would answer the door if I was naked? I thought to myself, but then realized it probably seemed that way since I was hiding my body behind the door. I opened the door all the way to prove that I was dressed and got up the nerve to question him.

"Mr. Green, were you a few doors down this morning walking around in your backyard?"

"Yeah, that was me," he answered casually. "I think your friend saw me and probably thought I was staring at her, but I wasn't, really. I was just looking for my keys. They fell out of my pocket somewhere along the way. I was hoping to find them. I just happened to look up and saw your friend. She was watching me." He pointed beyond where I stood.

I turned to see Kathy positioned behind me.

"I wasn't watching you. You were staring a hole right through me, and you know it! That's what made me turn around. Why do you wanna stand there and lie like that?" Kathy asked.

"I wasn't...Oh forget it. I just came up here to tell you both to come for dinner. I don't care if the two of you come or not."

Mr. Green turned in an attempt to walk away, but I stopped him.

"Now settle down. Both of you are getting all riled up over nothing. Mr. Green, we will be down in a few minutes. Thank you for taking the time to let us know."

"You're welcome, Miss. Uh, Miss?" He waited for me to fill in the blank.

"Jenny. Just call me Jenny. This is Kathy."

"Well, it's nice to meet you both. I'll be seeing you in the dining room in a few minutes. You are welcome to join me at the table on the far right side of the dining room, if you'd like."

Neither of us responded before he turned and headed down the hallway. I closed the door and saw Kathy was still in her defensive stance.

"Jenny, did you see his ears?" she asked.

"Yeah, they were different. But so what? Maybe he had some sort of accident. Maybe it's a birthmark or something."

"I guess you're right," Kathy agreed.

She softened her position. I could tell that the possibility that he was injured from an accident made her feel sorry for him all of a sudden.

She unknowingly stroked her own ears and then said, "Let's hurry and get downstairs before they send anyone else up here to get us."

CHAPTER NINETEEN

The chatter in the dining area sounded like buzzing bees. The atmosphere was one of a large family get together, as if everyone had known each other forever. The room was clean and decorated with pictures of moms, dads, and an old school house with children playing ball. The dinner was set up buffet style, so Kathy and I filled our plates and then looked for a place to enjoy our meal.

"Look, Jenny, there's Miss Spencer attending to tables on the other side. Maybe we should go sit there."

"Yes, let's do so," I agreed.

"Hey ladies, over here! There's plenty of room. I'm by myself," a male voice called out.

Kathy and I turned at the same time, looking in the direction of Mr. Green who was waving his arms to get our attention.

"What should we do?" Kathy leaned into me to whisper through her painted-on smile. "I don't want to sit with him. Do you?" she asked.

I painted the smile on too and waved back at him.

Through gritted teeth, I responded, "No, but we can't very well ignore him now, can we? Everyone in the room is already looking at us. I don't believe he's accustomed to using manners when out in public."

We walked over to his table as one unit like we were glued together at the hip.

"Hi, uh, Mr. Green was it?" I grinned courteously.

"Yes. Won't you ladies please join me?" He motioned to the two chairs opposite him.

"Yes, we would love to, Mr. Green."

I smiled and took a seat. I looked up at Kathy; yanked her down into the chair next to me, and she rolled her eyes at me like a bratty child.

"Please, call me Steve. My friends call me Steve. Oh, I know what both of you are thinking: We don't know this man from Adam's house cat, and we are definitely not his friends. Well, you will know more about me before our meal is over and, hopefully, change your minds." He smiled, took a sip of his water, and continued, "I am from the other side of Las Vegas. A little place called Death Valley. I'm an attorney and my clientele is comprised mostly of the criminally insane. I saw you both looking at my ears this afternoon. I could see you were wondering if I might be a real down-to-earth werewolf or something."

"No, honest, Steve, we thought perhaps you'd been in an accident or something. You see, we are nurses and are used to observing things of that nature. Aren't we, Kathy?"

"Well, uh, yes....yes, we are used to seeing things of that sort." Kathy fidgeted nervously in her chair.

The waitress walked over to our table and poured ice water into our waiting glasses. I was glad for the distraction. She topped off Steve's glass and left us to our uncomfortable conversation.

"Okay, let me clear this little matter up now. I was born this way. When my mother was pregnant with me, she was diagnosed with Grand Mal seizures. They put her on several medications. What you see is the result of several surgeries performed to correct the disfigurations caused by the medications. Pregnant women these days hardly even take vitamins, let alone the things they gave my mom when she was carrying me. But who knew those things back then? It's that simple, if you will. So, there you have the mystery of the man with the strange-looking ears." Steve took another sip of his water and sat back with his hands folded in front of him.

Kathy and I were silent. I made myself busy by placing my napkin on my lap, never once making eye contact with him. Kathy stared at her plate as she scooped mashed potatoes onto her fork.

"Oh, stop blushing," he added. "It's really not a big deal. I am used to people staring at me. In my profession, I see many, many people during the course of a day. Over the years, I've been stared at more than the Hope Diamond, I do believe."

"Do you still live in Death Valley or do you live in this area now, Steve?" I asked trying to change the awkward subject.

"No, I am actually here for a consult regarding one of my cases. I will be in town for a

152

few days. I always stay at this bed and breakfast. Do you ladies live here?"

"No," we replied in unison.

"What brings you two to this little town? Business perhaps?"

Steve smeared butter on his roll. Kathy continued eating so she could avoid the conversation. I guessed I was the only one left to respond.

"No, not at all. We're traveling. You know how it is when you want to try out new things in new places. We wanted to discover life in the big city, so we're on our way." I smiled and took a bite of my food hoping the interrogation wasn't going to last much longer.

"Oh. I see. So, you're Jenny with the red hair, if I recall." Steve smiled at me.

"Yes, I am Jenny, and the quiet one is Kathy." I pointed to my cohort who barely looked up from her plate.

"Well, now, Kathy with the black hat, why don't you join in the conversation and tell me what you think of moving to big city life." Steve leaned back waiting for her response.

Kathy took a sip of her drink. She paused before putting down her glass. He had just spoken to her like she was a child. I could tell that she was insulted.

I took a few more bites of my dinner knowing that I'd have to play referee momentarily. Kathy practically spat out her reply.

"Mr. Green. I think that's none of your business. Do you understand that?"

Steve's face turned red. He nervously pushed his glasses up the bridge of his nose and stammered out his response.

"Kathy, I humbly apologize for asking you that question in such a way that made you feel as though I was prying. I didn't mean to imply that at all. My fickle sister says that I am always trespassing into other folks' business. I mean nothing of the sort. So, please, quit calling me Mr. Green, and let's try to start again."

Steve wiped the sweat from his brow with his napkin. He took a long sip of water. Knowing Kathy was still seething, I answered for her.

"Forgive her, Steve. We are both exhausted from the mental strain of traveling. Tell me, where does your sister live, and what does she do for a living?"

His smile told me that he was relieved for the subject change in our conversation.

"She is a psychiatrist, but has recently retired. Well, she's retired from her practice, but for the past five years, she has been the manager of a place called Furnace Creek Inn."

"I've heard of that place. Isn't it the one built into the mountain side?" I asked.

"Yes, it is. It is exquisitely decorated and unique in its layout as well."

"That's an immense change for her, isn't it? I mean going from a psychiatrist to a hotel manager or something?"

"Yes, Jenny, it was a big switch in professional hats, so to speak. But there were some peculiar issues on her job, so she decided to retire early. The issues she had were serious in nature and loaded with legal ramifications, but I'm not at liberty to discuss them, of course."

"Oh my goodness, Steve, there's no way that we would expect such information to be divulged. Being nurses, we understand confidentiality better than the average person..."

I wiped my mouth with my napkin and placed it back in my lap. Kathy remained silent.

"Look, if you ladies are going in that direction or could take that route, I would be happy to call my sister tonight or tomorrow and make a reservation for the two of you. I think everyone should see it. You could stay there for a night or two. Shoot, I'll call her now if you ladies give me the okay." His eyes lit up with excitement.

"Steve, you don't even know us. Why would you do such a thing? We could be thieves or scam artists for all you know," I replied.

I wanted to believe he was being genuinely kind, but I had to be suspicious, for our own safety. Besides, Kathy was giving me the eye. I didn't think she wanted to go anywhere that this man suggested.

"Jenny, it's a long story, and it's about Kathy here. You see, she…"

Kathy interrupted, "It has nothing to do with me! How dare you, Mr. Green, if that's even your real name, try and imply that I….why we've never seen you in our lives!"

I dropped my fork onto the table.

"Kathy, for goodness sake, what in the world has come over you? Let the poor man finish his sentence." I was completely embarrassed by her rude behavior.

"That's okay, Jenny," he said to me and then looked at Kathy. "Forgive me, but I was just trying to say that you are the mirror image of my wife."

Kathy's jaw dropped open and her face flushed.

Steve continued, "She was correct when she said I was staring at her this morning. I *was* staring; but I was trying not to make it appear so conspicuous to you. You see, my wife disappeared a little over a year ago. I left for work one morning, and the house was empty that evening. She was gone. I've searched every city and town. I even hired a private detective, but he's come up empty handed every time. He'd think we had a good lead and off I'd fly to the town where she was supposedly seen. It was a big let down each time. When I saw Kathy this morning, I thought, 'This is it; that's her for sure.' There had to be a way for me to meet both of you in the dining room this evening. That's why I came to your room. I wanted to see her up close. Obviously she's not my wife. I realized that when I saw you upstairs. I'm sorry. I only have a glimmer of hope left, and I prayed that she was the end of my search. Kathy, I hope that I've relieved any anger that I've caused you or needless fear for that matter. I've meant you no harm."

Steve looked down dejectedly. Kathy didn't know what to say. Her voice cracked as she answered him.

"That's fine, Mr. Green. Uh, Steve. I understand. Thanks for explaining that and I apologize for being so abrupt with you this evening." She placed her napkin in her plate to signal the end of her meal. She turned to me and said, "Jenny, we better go upstairs and figure out where we're headed next."

She stood up from the table, put her purse on her shoulder, and I remained in my seat as I looked up at her.

"Well, Kathy, let's give Steve the go ahead to make the reservations for the inn and stay there for at least a day or so. We're not in a big hurry. It's out of the way, but, you know, it sounds really fascinating. What do you think?"

Kathy shrugged and answered, "That's fine."

"That's great! Alright ladies, I'll call my sister when I get back in my room. Do you need a map with directions to the inn?"

"No, I think we can find it. Kathy can read the map while I drive, and we'll watch for road signs that advertise it. We'll be fine. Thanks for everything, Steve." I stood and pushed in my chair. "Maybe we'll see you again someday. I sincerely hope you find your wife soon."

"Thank you Jenny and a good evening to both of you ladies. It's been my pleasure."

Steve politely stood up and I'm sure he watched us as we maneuvered our way out of the dining room. The stairway was dark and it felt eerie for some reason. We made our way back to our room with our own private fears. Once we were behind closed doors, I had to speak up about what had happened at dinner.

"I don't know that I've ever seen you so rude and as uptight as you were tonight. Your behavior embarrassed me, Kathy."

Kathy removed her earrings as she replied, "He made me angry this morning, staring so rudely at me. I never expected to be at dinner with him. Everything was just bottled up inside me."

The conversation replayed in my head as I changed into my pajamas. I guess I could understand why she was so upset with Mr. Green.

"Well, let's just get past all this and go to bed. I don't even want to watch the news tonight for fear we might see something negative. We'll get up early in the morning and start out for Death Valley. I'm kind of excited about it, aren't you?" I asked.

"Yes, I really am," Kathy answered with an almost convincing smile. She carefully folded her clothes and placed them in her luggage. "I'll pack today's paper in my suitcase and maybe while you're driving tomorrow, I can look over the job section around these parts to see what's offered."

"Okay," I replied, too mentally exhausted to say anymore. I brushed my teeth, Olayed my face, and couldn't wait to get into bed.

"All right, Jenny. Wake me in the morning if you get up before me. I want to get a cup of coffee before we leave." Kathy headed to the bathroom with her towel and toothbrush.

"Okay, will do. Goodnight."

"Goodnight, Jenny."

CHAPTER TWENTY

It was a beautiful day. Kathy and I were quiet, each inside our own musings. The highway was a long, winding path through nature as far as the eye could see. There was little traffic at this time of the morning, and it offered a feeling of peacefulness.

With Mom and Dad, I had always flown to Vegas and had never seen this part of Nevada. The cacti were in full bloom with the most beautiful, unusual-looking buds. I would have loved to stop and take pictures but decided that could wait until another time. Big balls of tumbleweeds seemed to be playing games with each other as they were rolled along by the wind. Every now and then a big ball would drift across the highway. Little critters that resembled rabbits would scamper by in a hurry. The desert wasn't enticing to me, but it was a different part of the world that one would enjoy seeing.

We'd been driving for about an hour when a sudden gust of wind came from nowhere and swirled about in a spiraling motion. It sort of mimicked a miniature tornado. It didn't seem to unnerve the other travelers ahead of us, so we assumed it was pretty normal for this area.

Kathy and I had gotten up early. We left without seeing anyone other than the owner of the bed and breakfast. When we paid our bill, she handed me an envelope from Steve Green. On the envelope, he had written a reservation confirmation number, a phone number, and his sister's name,

Miss Maggie Claire. It sounded like a comfortable name. I could see us sitting down with her and sipping tea, nibbling on fancy crumpets, and having a pleasant conversation.

The radio was playing music from the 40s era. Kathy and I had stopped earlier in the morning, bought a couple of Frappuccinos and muffins for breakfast. We knew that would tide us over until we reached Las Vegas. We both agreed that dining in Vegas would be a real treat plus an exciting experience.

"Hey, Jenny, turn the radio down and listen to this...'A new million dollar medical facility is scheduled to open next year in Boulder City, Nevada. It will be the first of its kind in the area. The facility will be headed up by professionals from several different states. Applications will be taken as early as next month.'"

"So, what's the big story there? What else does it say?"

"Well, nothing really; that's all it says." Kathy folded up the newspaper.

"So, what are you saying? I mean, do you think you want to live in Boulder City?"

Kathy looked at me quizzically.

"Well, no. I wasn't really thinking straight. We really don't need to live this close to California, I guess. Forget about it. I already have."

"Well, since you've gotten my attention now, does it list any of the founders?"

Kathy looked at the page in the paper again.

"No, it doesn't say a thing about any of that. Why, what difference does it make?"

"Oh, none whatsoever; I was just wondering that's all."

We drove in silence for several miles after that. I wasn't about to tell Kathy my ideas about the newspaper article. She would flip out; so I would let it slide for now.

"Okay, Kathy, turn the dial off the oldies station and find a boogie woogie station. Let's get things livened up here. Let's get down, girl. You know, like Thelma and Louise." I smiled with my tongue in my cheek.

"Really, Jenny? Tell me how we are going to boogie in this flippin' car. For Pete's sake, I sometimes wonder how you managed to get into the nursing profession with the way you've been acting lately."

Driving in the desert for too long must take its toll on your brain because we were both getting a bit punchy.

"Pete's sake? Tell me who in the heck is Pete, Kathy? You're always hollering about him, and I don't even know the man. Hey, Pete… C'mere, Pete. Kathy's calling you!"

"You've heard that saying as many times as I have! I've heard you say the same thing a few times. Don't act so juvenile, Jenny. Would you rather I learn to discuss things like a sailor? You know what they say about how sailors talk."

"Nah, I don't know what they say. I just wanna have some fun, and you won't even turn the radio to the magic station, you ol' stick-in-the-mud woman."

I couldn't help myself. I continued instigating. I was bored. Driving with the tumbleweeds for hours wasn't my favorite pastime.

"Look, Jenny, I really don't feel like trying to boogie in the car or whatever you are trying to do. You're driving the car and you need to concentrate."

"Just forget it, Kathy. We're almost in Vegas anyway. Have you given any thought to where you want to eat?"

"No, because I really don't know what's in Vegas. Let's look for their main street. I think they call it 'The Strip.' We can decide when we get there."

"Okay."

The traffic began to get heavier as we neared the outskirts of Vegas. It was a beautiful day, although we were used to seeing lush green grass, palm trees, and beach sand.

The mountains stood tall like a majestic back drop. The tops of the mountains seemed to be wearing caps of white as far as we could see.

"Look at that sign—five miles to Vegas." Kathy pointed. "We're almost there. I'm so excited. I've never been there. It will be a newly-made memory for us both. Maybe, if we ever get married and have children, we'll have some wonderful things to discuss about this adventure."

I wanted to say, "Yes, we can talk about when we worked at the hospital, stole organs from the living, and put computer chips in people's skulls." But instead I just bit my tongue and tried to behave.

"Whoa, Jenny, look at the traffic. It's almost bumper to bumper. Look at that large crater by the road there. I wonder what that's supposed to be. Look… oh my! Look at the big railroad sign that says 'Railroad Pass.' Oh, Jenny, it's a big casino. Look at the out-of-state cars. There's a car from Texas, one from Florida, even Mexico. I can't believe this."

Kathy was like a kid in a candy store. She was practically gushing as she pointed out our surroundings.

"I don't know why I'm acting like I've never seen bumper-to-bumper cars. I guess because I've lived in such a small town for my whole life. I'm just not used to this," she said apologetically.

"It's okay. I agree; it's exciting." I couldn't help but smile at her enthusiasm.

"Okay, we'll be coming into Henderson, Nevada. I think, according to the map, that's like the outskirts or something."

"Yes, Kathy, there it is. Henderson, Nevada. It looks like a pretty busy little town. I guess we better follow the map and go all the way to the main part of Vegas."

We were equally thrilled about the sights and seeing casinos scattered here and there. The tall buildings of downtown Vegas could be seen from where we were. It was absolutely breathtaking. We drove for a couple of miles when we saw fancy lights and bigger casinos: Circus Circus, the Mirage, Caesar's Palace, and the Venetian. It was like something from ancient Europe: Greek statues, beautiful fountains with colored water spraying beside gondola rides—just breathtaking! Casinos were lined up one next to the other like beautiful puzzle pieces that fit in perfection.

"I'm so excited! There are so many places to see. How can we possibly decide where to go first? I mean, just look at this place. As far as the eye can see it's like the state fair or a huge amusement park. It's unreal," I said. My eyes were darting from one thing to the next.

"I know, Jenny! I'm flabbergasted over the whole place. Look over there—the M&M store! Oh, look at the little M&Ms all over the casino. Let's go in there. Oh, let's spend the day… or maybe get a room for the night.

We can't just leave and not see some of the sights. We may never get back here again."

"I was thinking the same thing. I really can't think of any reason why we can't. I can easily reschedule our reservations at the inn for tomorrow night instead. Other than that, we aren't committed to being anywhere or to anything. No one is going to be hunting us down…at least not for a while," I added.

"Now, what's that remark supposed to mean?" Kathy asked.

"Just that if the team at the hospital starts missing us, they'll hunt us down if they think we are a threat to them in any way. That's all I meant. Settle down, Kathy. Let's plan to go to a show. Hey, how about the show at the Mirage? What are those famous magicians' names? Oh, I know: Siegfried and Roy. We can go to their show."

"Jenny, have you forgotten that Roy was attacked by one of his white tigers? They don't have that show anymore."

"Oh, that's right. I did read that somewhere a while back. Well, we'll do something else. Look over there, it's the New York, New York, and it has a roller coaster running around the whole outside of the bullding. I think it's attached to the building. Oh, my gosh, just look at that thing!"

There was too much to look at while driving by. I felt the need to stop so we could take it all in. This place was the perfect diversion for us.

"Let's drive back down the strip and get a room at the Holiday Inn. We'll change clothes, and then we can sightsee and have a nice dinner. How's that sound to you, Kathy?"

"Sounds like a plan to me. Let's go for it," she replied.

We checked into a room on the fourth floor. It was a picturesque view that offered so much more than we could have imagined.

As we toured the strip, we could hear music drifting out into the streets from the casinos. The sidewalks were covered with people of all sizes, shapes, and colors. We saw hair that stood straight up like spikes, with some colored every color of the rainbow, and there were even heads as bare as a baby's bottom. This was an exciting place with something different on every corner.

We bought souvenirs at several of our stops. We watched the fountains dance to music at the Bellagio and capped the night off with an amazing dinner at Caesar's Palace. We returned to our room completely exhausted from all the walking we had done, but the Vegas energy kept us awake later than usual.

"Oh, Jenny, what an exhilarating night this has been. The lights were like a thousand Christmas trees all in one setting."

Kathy was still mesmerized as she looked over the trinkets that she had purchased.

"I know, Kathy. I feel giddy like a teenager or something. The gondola ride was like riding through the channel inside the romantic city of Venice," I sighed.

This was one night we'd cherish forever. As we continued on our journey of escape from the things that lurked behind us, we were appreciative to have had the chance to visit Las Vegas. Hopefully the bliss of these unforgettable memories would carry us through as we faced the unknown things that lay ahead of us.

CHAPTER TWENTY-ONE

It was early morning. The sun had not yet peeped from its sky bed as we stepped into the empty elevator. We were hopeful we could make it to our next destination without any major problems.

Today we would drive to Furnace Creek and stay at the inn. I looked forward to meeting Mr. Green's sister, Maggie, and staying a day or so. I wondered why someone of her background was managing an inn. Something didn't seem quite right about it.

I had turned the news on last night to get a weather report while Kathy was in the shower. It seemed strange to hear the weatherman talking so seriously about rain and its impending dangers. I had given no thought to it until this morning when I heard it again. The forecaster said that it had been raining off and on all night. Kathy and I hadn't heard anything. We'd slept like logs.

We stepped off the elevator and headed toward the reservation desk.

"You ladies are leaving us after one night?" the man behind the reception desk asked.

"Yes, we have a few days of traveling to do before we get to our destination," I replied with a frown.

"Were your accommodations suitable?" he asked.

"Oh yes, I would say very much so. I hope someday in the future we can take a trip back and spend more time."

"Great. The bellman will have your luggage out front by the time they pull your car around. Have a safe trip and do come back," he added.

"Thank you. Have a great day!" Kathy exclaimed.

We walked outside to wait for our car. The air was thick and muggy. The clouds were rolling in like dark splotches of smoke. The wind was blowing hard. Rain was falling in light drizzles.

"My stars, Jenny, look at the clouds. It's like the wind is bringing black smoke from a huge fire and dumping it all around here," I groaned.

"I know. The palm trees are swaying, but not in a good way."

"Your car awaits, ladies. I do hope you had a memorable time. Did you win big enough at the casinos to want to come back and visit us again?" the valet driver asked.

"No, we didn't gamble, but the shopping is enough of a reason for us to come back." Kathy flirted.

The valet driver's eyes twinkled as he opened the passenger door for Kathy and she gracefully slid into her seat. After closing her in, he walked around to the driver's side and opened the door for me as well. Before closing the door he paused and said,

"Now you ladies be careful. Where are you headed from here, if you don't mind my asking?"

"We're going to Furnace Creek for a day or so," Kathy answered as she leaned across me.

"Hey, maybe you can give us directions to the highway we need to take from here. Have you heard of Furnace Creek?" I asked.

"Sure I've heard of Furnace Creek, Death Valley, and Scotty's Castle. You can't live here most of your life and not have heard of it, been to it, or know someone who's been there." He gave Kathy a quick wink.

Though the directions were for me, since I was driving, he gazed at Kathy the whole time he was speaking. She gleamed, batted her eyelashes, and nodded; as if she was mentally recording his every word.

"Okay, from here, you take a right when you pull out of the parking lot, go maybe 25 miles down, give or take a couple, and you'll see the sign that says Death Valley. After you get to that sign, you'll see a small gas station, makeshift grocery store and a couple of road signs. That's where you need to turn off for Death Valley, Furnace Creek, and all of those tourist attractions. You can find it easily. But, let me warn you about something..." He paused for effect as his face changed from flirtatious to one of concern. "It has been raining all night. There are flood notices going out in that area as we speak. The farther you drive toward Death Valley, the lower the altitude; it's very dangerous. My suggestion would be for you ladies to stay here in town tonight, at least until this rain blows over."

Huh! I see why he'd suggest such a thing. Sorry Kathy, we're not staying here so you can go out on a date.

"We really do appreciate all of your help, but I think we'll be okay. We're aware of the things that we need to be aware of, and you have updated us. I saw a few weather suggestions last night on the news. I think we'll be okay. Don't you think so, Kathy?"

I turned to see her reaction.

"How do I know, Jenny? I've seen nothing nor have I heard anything until this morning. You could've at least filled me in on what was happening with the weather. But, I guess we'll be fine. Rain is rain no matter where you are. Right?"

She looked to the guy for an answer.

"No ma'am. Rain is not just rain when it happens here, but do as you wish. You will anyway. Have a good life," he scoffed. As he closed my door, he waved us off and walked away.

"What's biting on his butt, do you suppose?" Kathy wondered suddenly turned off by his rudeness.

"I think he's concerned about what they call flash floods in these parts. In the desert, I could see where that could be a real serious issue, especially in low areas.

"Or, maybe he's just mad 'cause he won't have a date tonight," I mumbled.

About that time, we both let out a scream. A bolt of lightning cavorted across the sky like a cannon ball of fire. It gave me the willies. It seemed like an omen of some kind; like something or someone was trying to warn us that maybe we should stay at the hotel.

As I pulled out of the hotel entrance, Kathy asked, "Do you think we better wait like the guy suggested?"

"Nah, I think if we are cautious and stay alert to the conditions we'll be fine. We'll see what's going on as we get closer to the turn off. Stop worrying, Kathy. We've been okay this far. We'll be okay now." I tried to reassure her.

The clouds continued to hover over us like a giant blanket of gloom, but I was determined not to let this send us into some ridiculous frenzy. Besides, we were level-headed professionals and had enough sense to respond in the toughest of situations, and this was no different.

We rode for another thirty miles just looking out the window and staring at the mountains. The lightening continued to blaze the sky intermittently. Neither one of us said a word when drops of rain splattered on the windshield. I guess we thought if we said nothing about it we'd be fine, and it would stop because we wished for it to stop.

"There's the sign." Kathy pointed. "It says,

'Turn right to see Death Valley, Scottie's Castle, and Furnace Creek Inn.' This is our turn. The inn is 183 miles from here."

"Okay, let's see. There's the gas station just like the guy told us, and I do want to stop before we start toward Death Valley. We need to fill the gas tank, check the radiator and hoses, and do whatever we need to make sure the car is running well. Oh, get this Kathy, I read a brochure at the hotel that says if you break down in the desert, you most likely will die of heat or wild coyote attacks. It mentioned the flash flooding thing too. It advised anyone in that position to seek higher ground immediately; so I wouldn't want the car to break down for any reason. I think it's a pretty desolate road, and we shouldn't take unnecessary chances."

"Great. I really needed to know that stuff now. Thanks a lot, Jenny!"

Kathy crossed her arms. I ignored her childish pout.

"I'll see about the car. You go in and get us some coffee, maybe some chips or something to eat, too. I guess we should've had a piece of toast this morning, because I'm a bit hungry. Aren't you?" I asked.

"Now that you've mentioned it, yes, I am. I'll go get us some food so we can fend off the coyotes or so we don't have to resort to cannibalism or anything like that while we're stuck in the desert." She smirked as she got out of the car.

Soon we were driving along a narrow road

that seemed to wind downhill between huge mountains stacked high with large boulders. The sun was nowhere to be seen, and the rain was getting a little heavier. We passed a few cars, which I was very glad to see. I was beginning to feel jittery. I didn't dare let Kathy know.

I turned the windshield wipers on high and noticed that the wind was beginning to whip up. I asked Kathy to turn the radio back on hoping it would take my mind off of being out here in the middle of nowhere, in the rain, and with this overwhelming feeling of impending doom.

"Stop! Stop, Jenny!" Kathy shouted. "What are those things running across the road?"

I braked as I saw what she was referring to and the car slid as it slowed. I couldn't come to a complete stop even if I wanted to.

"Dogs, just some sort of dogs, it looks like, running in a pack." I tried to make out what I thought I was seeing.

"Do something, Jenny. Hurry, you have to stop the car!" Kathy was insistent.

"And what good will that do? We have to keep going. That's all we can do. Hold on and just be quiet," I commanded.

"But, Jenny, look out there. There's a whole group of them. You can't just run over them. Stop!"

"Kathy, for crying out loud, I am not trying

to run over them. I am trying to scare them into running into the desert. Sit back and just be quiet!"

I maneuvered the car slowly but steadily down the road. It took what seemed like an eternity before the pack of dogs or coyotes realized they'd better move or get hit. I looked over at Kathy who was sitting with her face cupped in her hands. Perspiration beaded on my upper lip. My heart was pounding hard in my chest. I had never seen such a thing in my life and certainly had never driven into something like this. I prayed I never would again.

"Kathy, it's okay. You can raise your head. Look, nothing happened. If you think for one moment that this didn't upset me, you're dead wrong. It's a long way out here, we're alone in the desert, and it's raining hard. We are going to have to pull over somewhere in the next few seconds. It's getting too dangerous."

Then the rain started coming down even harder and it was blowing in sheets. I remembered what the news anchor said about the dangers of flash floods. I admitted to myself that leaving the hotel had been a bad decision.

I could see a car coming toward us with its lights flashing. It was an emergency vehicle with a light swirling on top like a police car. I heard a male voice shouting into a loud speaker, "Get to higher ground quickly. Please get to higher ground."

He passed us yelling something about waves of water rushing in our direction and that we needed to get out of the car immediately to seek higher ground. I panicked, not knowing what to do. I saw a van pulled off to the side of the road. It looked as though the passengers had deserted it. I was frightened. Others had evacuated, and Kathy and I were stranded on the road. I looked over at Kathy who, by this time, had a death grip on the door handle. The rain was coming down so hard now that the windshield wipers were no longer able to keep the window free of the deluge.

Suddenly, I saw it coming. The water rushed toward the car. It was coming straight for us. I knew there was no way of getting out of the car now, nor out of the way of the racing water. We were going to die, and there were so many things that I should have done. Fragments of my life were swirling through my head as fast as the water that waited to swallow us in its murky silence.

I yelled at Kathy to hold on tight. I put my foot on the brake and held the steering wheel as tightly as I could. The muddy water mixed with debris hit us like a giant sledge hammer. As it pummeled us from all sides, the car was pushed around like a miniature matchbox car. I looked at Kathy. She was as white as a ghost and wasn't saying a word. She looked like a statue made of concrete. Sickness swept over me as the car moved like a ship on a rough sea. The water rose to the doors and the floor was filling up quickly. I felt a jolt that threw both of us toward the windshield. We'd hit something. The car came to a halt.

It was quiet, and the rain slowed considerably. The windows were covered in mud.

There wasn't a clearing that would allow us to see outside. I didn't know what to do. What if we were on the side of a drop off or something? The water had taken the car in all directions. I sat still; too afraid to open the door or roll down the window. Suddenly, I heard a loud knock on the front window. Kathy let out her first scream as a sign that she still felt some sort of emotion.

"Hello in there. Can anyone hear me? I am here to help you. It's okay. I am the ranger from Scotty's Castle. Hello. Please respond so I can help you," announced the man's voice.

"Yes! Oh, my God, yes. We're in here. We're okay, I think. Can you open the door? Can you please open the door and get us out of here?" I pushed on the door frantically as I pulled the handle, but the door wouldn't budge. "Hey, we can't get out. Oh, please don't let us die in here. The door won't open. Are you there? Hello?!" I called out again, desperate to hear his response.

"Ma'am, please calm down. I will get you out. How many of you are in there?" the muffled voice asked.

"Two. There are two of us. I'm Jenny and my friend Kathy is here. Can you get us out of this car?" I continued my unsuccessful attempts to open the door; it was no use.

"Yes, just hang on and don't panic. The worst is over, and you've survived it. Don't worry if the car shakes a bit. You're in a safe place. I need to pry your door open. It's caked up pretty thick with mud. The passenger door is blocked by a hummock of dirt. You'll both need to climb out on the driver's side. Now, hold on while I loosen your door."

The jarring startled us both. Kathy started shaking as though she had severe chills.

"Kathy, settle down. We're going to be okay."

I reached out to hold her hand. Kathy took a quivering breath as a tear escaped from her eye.

"Okay, Jenny. I'm fine. God only knows, but I think I am fine. I thought we were about to die, and I wondered what would happen if no one found us for days. I'll be okay."

I hugged my friend over the center console. We had been through so much together, both good and bad. She sniffed and let her tears flow onto my shoulder.

"Okay, ladies, one more yank at the door and you'll be outta there."

A loud creaking sound was followed by a lot of shaking, and the door finally opened. I tried to get out and fell back onto the seat. Again, I tried, and my feet hit the mud and water. I grasped the hand of the kind ranger, and I managed to stand up. His outstretched hand reminded me of the hand of God. As I turned to look at Kathy, the ranger thought I was stable and let go of my hand. I lost my balance and fell onto layers of muddy water and rocks, cutting my hands and legs.

"Oh, miss, I'm so sorry that I let you slip. Here, take my hand, and let me get my arm around your waist. Here, now let me take you to the van and get you settled, and then I'll come back to get your friend."

His voice was so comforting. He nodded to Kathy to reassure her that he'd be right back.

I struggled to my feet then he assisted me into the waiting van. The mud and water came up above our ankles.

"What about our car? What happens to our car and our things?" I asked.

"We'll pull it on the tow truck. I have already called, and they'll be here as soon as they can. Some of the roads are closed so it'll take a bit longer for them to get to us than it normally would. Once the tow truck is here, they'll pull you to wherever you're going, within reason." Once I was seated in the van he said, "Well, let's get your sister out of the car and be on our way."

I probably didn't need to answer, but for some reason, I did.

"Oh, she's not my sister. She's a good friend and a nurse, like me. Her name is Kathy. I am Jenny."

The ranger's caring eyes warmed me to the core. He saved us and I couldn't have been more grateful to him. He was our hero.

"Alright, Jenny, I'll get Kathy to the van, and both of you girls will be on your way in no time. You can get a good, hot bath and get this mess off you. Then we can fix those cuts and bruises you have there, and try to relax after such a horrible ordeal. We've had reports of deaths during this thing, and I think you girls need to know how lucky you are."

It wasn't long before Kathy and I settled into the ranger's van. The rain finally stopped and the driving conditions improved tenfold. The tow truck that would retrieve our car was en route. We decided to leave everything in it except for our toiletries and pajamas. I assumed the car was going to need many repairs. It had tons of mud all over it and dents in the sides and on the hood. I hoped the engine wasn't ruined. I looked down and there was mud on my pants up to my knees. I didn't care. We were alive, and that was all that mattered.

We rode the next few miles listening to the ranger talk about the floods he had worked, the numerous deaths that were related to floods, and other types of deaths related to the storm. I knew it wasn't a place I'd ever visit again. We said little to each other as we continued the drive. Kathy tried to make small talk, as she felt it polite to interject a word every now and then, but neither of us really wanted to talk. We drove another hour before pulling up to the most beautiful place one could imagine. It was like an image out of a picture book of the most unique places one would ever see. Here in the side of the mountain was a hotel that looked as though someone had carved out each piece before placing it cozily inside the rocks and boulders. The mountain held it like a glove. I couldn't believe my eyes.

"Okay, ladies. Here we are. I'll take you in so you can settle into your room. I'll get your things out of your car and send them to your room as soon as the tow truck gets here."

The inn was bustling with guests. We weren't sure if they had gotten stranded due to the storm or if the place stayed full all year round. There was an attractive blonde lady behind the desk. She was deep in conversation with someone. The park ranger waited until she was finished and then he made himself known.

"Hey, honey!" The ranger leaned over the desk and kissed the blonde on the cheek. "I found the two nurses that your brother told you were coming. This is Jenny and her friend Kathy. They were caught in the flood while on their way here. They are lucky to be alive. Ladies, meet my fiancée, Miss Maggie Claire. She'll get you settled. I've got things to do and reports to finish. You ladies have a good evening and welcome to Furnace Creek Inn."

"Kathy and I don't know how to thank you for all that you've done for us. How can we ever repay you? You literally saved our lives today and we don't even know your name!"

We took turns shaking his hand and hugging him.

"You owe me absolutely nothing. I was just doing my job. Oh, and the name is Frank. Frank O'Hara. It's been a pleasure meeting you both."

He tipped his hat to us, winked at his fiancée, and waved as he left us in her care.

Miss Claire walked around the desk to greet us with a hug.

"Well, it is so good to see you both. My brother called a couple of evenings ago to get things set up for you. I wanted to call him today to see if you had left yet, but the phone lines are all down. Helicopters from the media and the National Park Service have been flying over various parts of the area assessing the damage. I am sort of stuck out here for now; although they assured me that phone service would be restored in a couple of days. Hey, enough dreary discussions. I imagine you ladies are ready for a room and a nice, hot bath."

"Yes, Miss Claire, we are about ready to crumple, I think. Aren't we, Kathy?"

Kathy nodded in agreement.

"Yes, we are. This has been one nerve-racking day. You would think nurses could withstand anything, but I think this has almost whipped us. I have never seen nature's wrath quite like I did today."

"I'm sorry you had to endure this sort of thing on your first visit with us, but we never know when nature's going to pay us an unforgettable visit. You really are lucky to be alive and able to talk about it. There are numerous death reports coming in as we speak. The police scanner reports numerous roads washed out, massive chunks of asphalt jutting up from the mud, bodies buried alive in their vehicles."

She stopped speaking as she processed the thought of it all.

Kathy and I knew those dead bodies could have easily been ours.

Maggie added, "Please forgive me. I shouldn't be telling you this after what you have experienced today, but I am thankful you're safe. It has been devastating. Please, come with me. I'll take you to your room. I have reserved a large suite, two king-size beds, and all of the amenities of home. It's more like a small apartment, and I think you'll find it to your liking."

"I'm sure we will," I replied.

Ms. Claire took my arm and led us to our room. She opened the door and invited us in for a quick tour.

"There's a menu on the dresser. Just call if you decide to order. Extra towels and pillows are in the hall closet over here."

"Thank you, Miss Claire. Thank you so very much," Kathy said.

"Oh, please. Don't call me that. Just call me Maggie. That's all anyone here calls me. I was Miss Claire for far too many years. It came with the position, but now, it's the casual life for me."

"Yes, I believe your brother told us you had been a psychiatrist for many years."

"I was, and guess I still am, but I am not

184

practicing in a big office somewhere or a hospital setting. I miss that part of my life, but this position with the inn allows me to talk with people, and sometimes they will come to me with mental issues that concern them."

"Did you have a large practice in a big city?" Kathy asked.

"Yes, I did. I was also on the board of directors at one of the biggest hospitals in Pennsylvania. I really loved the intervention with in-patient clients. And I really enjoyed being included in the decision making about newly-developed programs, but all of that had to come to an end."

Maggie nervously fixed the pillows on the couch as she talked about what was obviously a difficult job for her to leave.

"May we ask why you left such a prestigious position to come to a desolate place like this? Well, maybe it's not desolate, but being out in the middle of the desert is pretty desolate to most people."

I pried maybe a little too much. Her demeanor changed pretty quickly.

"Let's just say I had my reasons. Here is your key. I need to be going. I have tons of work waiting in my office. Order your dinner whenever you feel like eating. The front desk has a number directly to my place should you need to call." She headed to the door, but paused when she got there.

She turned and asked, "By the way, since you are both nurses who worked in a small town hospital, why did you choose to leave?"

Hmm, which one of us is brave enough to answer this one? I wondered. Of course, it had to be me.

"Oh, well we uh, I became dissatisfied with the hum-drum routine. So, Kathy and I discussed it, and we both decided to strike out for the big city."

"Jenny, why…"

"Kathy, your cell phone is ringing. You better answer it."

I walked to the door to break up the discussion. I wasn't about to tell a stranger that we were caught up in some organ stealing business.

"Thank you, Maggie, for all you've done. It's been so nice meeting you, and I am sure we'll see you tomorrow."

She shook my hand and smiled.

"Nice meeting you, too. Good night, ladies."

I closed the door behind her and turned to find Kathy in my face.

"Why in the world did you lie to her, Jenny? And why in the world did she change the subject when you asked her why she left her old job?"

I skirted around her to get away. I was really needing some alone time.

"I have no idea, but I do know this: I don't know her and I'm not about to divulge to her what's going on with us. I do know she seemed very uncomfortable when we asked about her job situation. I think she is hiding something, and we may find out the hard way. I feel very strange about the whole thing, and her demeanor suddenly changing like that."

My mind was on overload. Today had taken its toll on me, and it was all I could do to keep from sobbing. I wanted nothing more than to take a long, hot shower to wash off all evidence of what we went through in Death Valley. *Now I know why they call it that!*

"Oh, gracious, Jenny, this place is like a full-size apartment. This must be one of the highest-priced rooms available."

She walked back into the bedroom where I remained stuck in a daze.

"What's wrong? You look as if you're about to cry."

"Huh? No, I'm okay. I apologize. I've been listening to you, but reality just reared its ugly head. I am so aware of how close we came to death today. I'm going to bed. I can't think of eating a thing. You order something if you wish, but a nightcap and a sleeping pill are what I need right now. Don't worry about me. I'm tough, but today was a bit much on top of everything else. We'll talk tomorrow, Kathy. Good night."

"I understand. Tomorrow will be a better day, Jenny."

I nodded and tried to grin, but all I could think about was washing off the muck that covered me, getting into bed, and closing my eyes...

CHAPTER TWENTY-TWO

The noise roused me from a deep sleep. It sounded like boulders dropping into our bedroom. I didn't hear Kathy stirring and wondered how she could sleep through it. I jumped up and ran to the window. I saw a huge boulder fly past the window into a pile that lay just beyond our cabin. Bucket trucks were everywhere. I had forgotten about the debris from the flash flooding. The news had elaborated on the widespread damage in and around Death Valley. As I stood looking at the pile, I was reminded of the nightmarish flooding of the previous day and the fact that Kathy and I were almost killed.

Suddenly a knock at the door reeled me back into reality. I wondered who it could be since no one knew where we were. It was probably Maggie. I felt relieved thinking that surely it was her. I headed for the door when the phone rang. I decided to let the phone ring and get the door. A bellboy was standing there with a sullen look on his face. He looked as though he'd been inside his own nightmare. He handed me an envelope and quickly left before I had a chance to thank or question him. I couldn't tell who the letter was for. There was nothing written on it. The postmark was smudged and muddy. It must have gotten messed up during the flooding. I decided I would open it, and if it was for Kathy, then I would give it to her. The phone stopped ringing. Kathy hadn't come out of her room. The envelope in my hand caused my heart to pound like a set of drums. It was probably from Maggie's brother.

I opened the envelope enough to see a note taped across the top with blue tape. The trembling began slowly from the inside out. How foolish of me to carry on in this way. Kathy would behave like this, not me. I pulled the tape off while trying not to tear the note. There it was staring back at me. My breath was hiding deep within me, unwilling to cooperate. I wondered if this was how it felt to asphyxiate. I managed to get up from the couch and ran to Kathy's room. I swung the door open so hard it slammed against the wall. She sat straight up in the bed and yelped.

"Kathy, you must get up. Now! Hurry! We have to get ready to leave this place as soon as possible." I yelled frantically.

"What's wrong with you? What happened?"

"Read this note, and you'll see. Get up. We have to go."

Kathy took the note, staring in horror at the words. They seemed to leap out at her with a foreboding presence as she read them aloud.

"Jenny, did you really think that you could get away from Dad and me? We'll be seeing you soon, real soon, dear."

The color drained from Kathy's face.

"Oh, Jesus, help us. How did they find us? What are we going to do? Have they followed us here?"

She stumbled out of bed and quickly changed out of her pajamas.

"I don't know, Kathy. I swear I don't know. You know I didn't tell them. I told you back when we found out about their involvement with The Group that as far as I was concerned they were already dead. C'mon, we've got to get downstairs and talk to Maggie. She'll know if someone has been here looking for us. Maybe she knows who sent this note too. Okay, we must calm down," I said trying to assuage myself.

Fortunately our luggage was delivered before we fell asleep last night. My head was spinning like a top. Questions were darting like arrows without a place to land. I had no answers and could only hope Maggie Claire could tell us enough to put some sort of picture together. The one thing I felt strongly about was leaving this place as soon as possible.

"Let's go to breakfast, find Maggie, and ask her to join us. We'll act as casually as possible. She mustn't know how upset we are."

"All right, Jenny, I know you're right. She must not suspect that we are running. We can't afford to trust anyone, not anyone at all."

We walked into the dining area. Every table was full. Finally, an elderly couple got up from the table by the window. We were headed in that direction when I heard a male voice calling our names. It was Maggie's brother, Steve. How in the world had he made it here so soon when he was supposed to be working on a murder case? I felt uneasy as I tried to smile and pretend things were fine. I looked at Kathy, who had pasted a smile on her face, although she looked like someone in a hypnotic state.

"Hey, Steve, we thought you were tied up on a murder case. We didn't expect to see you here," I said.

"Uh, no, we didn't. My goodness, this is quite a surprise," Kathy added.

"Well, ladies, I finished what needed to be done and decided to drive down. I had a few problems getting through some of the roads though. It looks like a bomb went off in these parts. I had to detour several miles out of the way. I tried to phone Maggie, but I couldn't get through to the inn. Anyway, I'm here now." He smiled as if we'd be happier to see him.

"Well, uh, won't you join Kathy and me for brunch?" I asked, trying to be polite.

"I'd love to! Have you seen Maggie this morning?" His eyes quickly scanned the room.

"No, we haven't. We just walked in when you saw us. I'm sure she's here somewhere close by. She's probably busy with all of the work crews coming and going."

We headed for the empty table together. Steve held out our chairs for each of us to sit. He took an extra chair from a nearby table for himself and sat down with a menu.

"Once we've ordered and we're waiting to be served, I'll go find her," Steve said.

"Sounds good, I think I'll start with a cup of coffee. What about you, Kathy?"

"I'll have hot tea," Kathy replied.

I could tell she was not happy that we were dining with Steve Green again. *What was I supposed to do? Ignore the guy?* We were reviewing our menus when Maggie came around the corner from the registration desk. She appeared to be disturbed about something and didn't look up. A few seconds passed then Maggie put something in her pocket. She looked in our direction and smiled, then headed toward us.

"Good morning, ladies. I see my brother has taken control of you already." She looked at Steve with a sweet little smirk.

"Oh, now, Maggie, don't scare my new friends off with your comments. Of course, now that you mention it, I wouldn't mind such a thing. What red-blooded American man wouldn't wish to control a few pretty women? Hmm, I better hush while I'm still in everyone's good graces."

Kathy fidgeted uncomfortably in her seat. Surely she was thinking what I was thinking.

"Steve, I'm sure these ladies don't find you that amusing. What brought you here this week anyway? I thought you were on a big murder case."

Maggie straightened the sugar packets on our table.

"I was, but I was able to tie up the loose ends, and here I am; at least for now," Steve clarified.

After the way Steve raved about his sister, I would have thought she'd be happy to see him. However, I got the feeling she was as suspicious with his arrival as we were.

"Why didn't you at least call and let me know you were coming?" Maggie asked.

"I tried, Maggie. I really tried several times, actually, but the lines were down. It's a miracle that I'm here. There are power lines lying across roads, huge boulders scattered everywhere, and roads gone. I had to detour way out of the way and then I got lost. Look, why don't you tell us what's good for brunch, and never mind the rest of the whys and hows. I need to make a quick business call, and then I'll be ready to eat. I'm starved."

Maggie eyed him but didn't respond. Instead she turned to us and asked, "How about it, ladies? Would you like me to go into the kitchen and have the chef prepare my special along with some of our newest side items?"

"That would be so kind of you, Maggie, but, please don't go to any extra trouble for us. We are easy to please," I insisted.

"Oh, it's no bother at all. I really enjoy doing this for special guests. I'll be back in a jiffy."

Maggie left, and Steve excused himself to make a phone call. Kathy quietly stared out the window. I had pondered the many questions I had about the note I'd received. How could Mom and Dad find me? What was going to happen next? There seemed to be no answers as I wondered what lay ahead in our future.

"Jenny, what are we going to do about these people? We've allowed total strangers to come into our lives. People we don't even know. Why are these things happening to us? Why?"

Evidently, Kathy was preoccupied with the note as well.

"Well, they aren't really a problem for us. I honestly feel this was a happenstance situation. They are both very educated professionals and seem sincere for the most part.
I think that you and I have become too paranoid since this nightmare began."

Steve startled us into silence when he returned to the table.

"All right, ladies, things are under control for the time, and I am famished. How about you two?"

"Why, yes, Steve, we could eat. I'm sure Maggie will have something delightful prepared. So tell me, how long will you be staying here with Maggie?"

I unfolded my napkin and placed it on my lap hoping the food would arrive soon.

"That depends on what you mean. Do you mean at the inn or in and around Death Valley?"

"Just here at the inn," I replied.

"Probably three to four days. Why? Can I assist you with something?"

"No, my goodness, gracious, no. I was just curious. I had no reason for asking, and I don't mean to be prying. I'm sure that Maggie is more than happy to see you."

I fixed my placemat and took a sip of my water.

"Maggie and I are very close. We have always enjoyed the same things. Since our parents passed away, we have no other relatives, really, so I try to come see her when business permits me to get away for a few days. Speaking of Maggie, here she comes now. Great!"

The waiters trailed Maggie with a large platter holding a wide selection of brunch dishes.

"I hope your palates and appetites are ready. I think you are going to be most pleasantly surprised at what we have selected for you."

Maggie presented each of us with multiple plates.

"It looks scandalously delicious, dear sister." Steve grabbed his fork and knife and was ready to devour.

"How can we ever repay you, Maggie? Maybe when Kathy and I get settled, you can come visit us. We would welcome an opportunity to repay some of your graciousness."

"Oh, that won't be necessary. Just let me know how things taste. I've been trying to gather opinions about these specialty items, so I can approach the owners for new menus along with a few other needed changes around this place."

With quite a bit of prodding, Maggie decided to sit and join us. Brunch was quiet except for the occasional joke by Steve. He said he needed to spice things up a bit for us. Kathy and I said very little. Maggie told us about her engagement to our ranger hero, Frank, and all about how they met. The dining area was now empty except for an older couple across the room. They seemed to be arguing. Maggie left the table to take a phone call and was making her way back.

"Maggie, I was wondering if we could ask you a couple of questions regarding your position at the hospital."

My inquiry caused Maggie to stop herself from clearing our plates. She sighed, placed the pile of dishes in the center of our table, and sat down.

"Yes, I suppose so, Jenny; however, I'm not at liberty to divulge much to you. I know you understand. Professional ethics and confidentiality are of utmost importance. I can't afford to seek counsel for a lawsuit. You know this better than anyone."

"Yes, of course, I understand." I nodded and continued, "Let me start with an envelope that I received this morning. It was brought to our room by one of your bellboys. I need to know how it arrived. Neither of us has family, and we didn't tell anyone that we were coming to the inn. So we are very curious about how this note arrived. Could you tell us who delivers the mail out here?"

Maggie's look changed from exasperated to one of concern as she replied, "No, I really can't say, other than the local postal service. They deliver all mail by helicopter when floods close the road. A load of mail was brought in this morning. We always place it in the mail slots designated for each room. I can't tell you any more than that." She paused and then added, "We've had cases where Vegas Red Cross would send emergency personnel out, but that usually involved the death of a guest's family member or significant other. Generally those recipients had people who knew their whereabouts though. Is something wrong?"

"Well, no, not at all, Maggie. Everything is fine. We were just curious." I tried to sound convincing.

"But Jenny, you said that we ..." Kathy interjected.

"It's really not an issue, Kathy." I cut her off. "Remember the discussion we had this morning? Let's not worry these gracious people with that sort of thing."

"Oh, okay. Please excuse me, Maggie. I get the cart ahead of the horse more often than not," Kathy apologized.

Maggie and Steve glanced at each other. Our behavior was definitely confusing to them.

"Maggie, you told us that you left your last position, which was one of prestige. I don't mean to pry, but like you, Kathy and I have multiple reasons for the changes we are making, as well. I don't wish to be inappropriate in my questions, but I would like to inquire about the hospital's leadership."

"Are you inquiring about the hospital administrator?"

"Yes, I was wondering if you could give me a name." I stared at her hoping for a response that would be different from the one I feared.

"I suppose there's no harm in giving out the particulars about the hospital administrator. He's well known over several states. His name is Dr. Kenalog. Do you perchance know him, or have you met him in your medical dealings?"

Kathy gasped when she heard his name. She jumped up from the chair and ran toward our room. I felt as though someone had placed his hands around my throat and was squeezing the life out of me. I could feel my heart hammering as each beat echoed stronger and louder inside my head. I felt the color leave my face as I struggled to catch my breath. I was vaguely aware that Steve had jumped up and ran around the table; he took my hand in his. I couldn't say a word.

"Jenny, are you alright? Tell me what to do. Are you sick? Maggie, run and find the first aid kit. I hope you have smelling salts."

"Steve, take me… take me to where…Kathy. I am going to fa…" I moaned.

Maggie retuned in a blink with a medical bag in her hand. She rummaged through and quickly opened a small container of smelling salts then held them under my nose.

"Okay, okay, that should do it. She's beginning to come around. Back up a little and give her some air," Steve suggested.

Though I was barely coherent, I sat up and interrogated them.

"Where's Kathy? Someone please tell me what happened. Did I pass out? Oh, God, no. Tell me this is a dream. This can't be happening to us."

"Jenny, please tell me, what in the world did I do or say that caused such drastic reactions from both you and Kathy? I don't understand. You asked me a question, and I answered it briefly. I am really lost as to what is going on now. I gave you a name, and you flipped out."

Maggie held a cold cloth to my face. I pushed her hand away and attempted to stand, but my feet wouldn't cooperate with me. I was trembling uncontrollably.

"Maggie, I need to ask you once more. What was the name you gave me? Please tell me once again the name of the hospital administrator."

My voice sounded raspy. I could barely hear the words coming out of my own mouth. It was like someone had just put me in a glass jar and placed a lid securely over me. There were two of Steve and Maggie. I struggled to maintain my upright position.

"Jenny, his name is Dr. Kenalog. Do you know him? Please, it is very important that you tell me this. If you do, I must know your connections with him. I must!"

I thought I would throw up on them at the very mention of his name. I held back my tears.

"I am fearful of saying anything to you regarding Dr. Kenalog. But if you know him, and I mean know him, then you may have the same concerns as I do."

Maggie's eyes widened. She shared some of my fear. *Does she know what we know about him?* I wondered.

"Jenny, I will put two and two together. I will answer both your questions and mine. Yes, I know all about his dealings, and that's why I left the hospital. I know without you telling me that you and Kathy left your hospital for the same reasons. We must talk candidly and try to come up with some kind of logical plan. I will show you something, but first I must tell you that I am in no way affiliated with him or The Group."

I gasped. *She knows about The Group!* I felt a sense of relief when I realized Kathy and I weren't alone in this, but the note we received that morning made the situation even more complex now. We were not the only ones in danger.

"Do you see this scar on the inside of my wrist?" Maggie moved her watch up to show me a mark. "Don't ask me anything. Save your time and energy. No, I am not one of them, but only because the chip failed due to improper handling and placement. I found a way to ensure that it could never be traced with what they called the Lasernator. I heard them speak of it quite by accident one day. I was preparing a report when I discovered that I had left some paperwork in Dr. Kenalog's office. I walked down the hallway at the north end of the hospital. This location was off limits to hospital traffic unless you had a special pass. I heard him on the phone talking with someone about the Lasernator.

"I'd had surgery on my hand previously for an unknown pain that was crippling my right arm, and I was unable to work because of it. I was x-rayed, and it was determined that I had severe nerve damage. I was in a skiing accident many years ago, and the damage was extensive on this side.

I visited a neurologist, and long story short, was referred for surgery. Dr. Kenalog was to do the surgery but told me he would be out of town so one of his colleagues would be doing it. I woke up some time later with what felt like a fire literally burning me underneath my skin. It felt almost like an electrical shock of some kind that kept pounding away in the area of the surgery. I couldn't see anything, but I could feel it.

"I had previously found out about some unorthodox procedures that were going on at the hospital. I pretended to go along with him, acting like something was wrong with me. The doctor who performed the surgery asked me if I suddenly had the urge to do things without thinking about it. I told him yes, although being in the mental health profession gave me a good working knowledge of how to play his game. I feared that a chip had been placed in my arm. I'd seen them place these gadgets in numerous donor tissues and surgery patients. Those tissues have been shipped all over the world, I suppose."

Of course! How stupid of us! They were implanting the donor parts with the chips as well! I hadn't thought about that before now. I knew that people were being implanted, but I didn't realize the organs that were being donated around the world were implanted as well.

Maggie added, "You're also probably wondering if I've been to their big meeting. I believe they call it a 'coming out meeting.'

"Yes, I have been to the nightmare with its stench of death. I acted as much like the others as I could. I mimicked their every move. I was only able to escape thanks to the help and persistence of my brother. Now, you know why I left and why I've tried to hide out here in this desolate wasteland. I know many people are walking around all over the USA implanted with chips. Now, it's time that you and Kathy tell me what the hell is going on with you. Are you part of their movement?"

Angered by hearing about what they did to her, I was able to find the strength to stand up. I pulled her out of the dining area, away from everyone, including Steve. We retreated to a hallway where I was able to respond to her without the fear of someone else hearing.

"I don't know where to begin. I must tell you first and foremost, that Kathy and I are running from them, too. We are not in on their evil scheme. I still don't understand why it's happening. The nightmare to end it all for us was the coming out meeting. That's where you fit in, Maggie. That note that came today was from my parents. They were at the coming out meeting. They are now part of The Group. Have they traced us here? If they have found Kathy and me, then that means you will be found, too. What are we going to do? We've all got to get out of here."

I was grabbing onto her arm as tears flooded my eyes. I felt so sorry for everything.

She was safely hidden here for however long it has been, was happily engaged to be married, and now, thanks to us, she would be found.

She looked over her shoulder as a couple turned out of the dining area to walk toward us down the hallway.

"Jenny, first of all you need to go check on Kathy, and then let's meet back in my office. We'll compile all of our facts together. We must have privacy. No one must hear our conversations. We are in serious danger and we need to come up with a plan."

Her stance was strong. She was obviously determined, unwavering, and she wasn't going to give up without a fight. I agreed, trying to absorb some of her courage.

"Okay. I'll get Kathy and meet you in your office, but I would first like to ask you about your brother, Steve. So he, I mean, you said he helped you. So he has knowledge of all of this?"

"Yes, he was there for my surgery, and he knew what they had done to me. I have been working with him on this for a year now," she whispered.

The couple passed us and continued down the hall to their room. There was nothing left to say. We went our separate ways. I hurriedly walked toward our room.

It felt like someone's eyes were watching my every move, yet I knew there wasn't a place for anyone to hide. I couldn't shake the jittery feeling that enveloped me like a glove.

CHAPTER TWENTY-THREE

The things that I'd learned from Maggie blew me away. I returned to the room to find Kathy had fallen asleep on the couch. *How could she sleep at a time like this?* The television was playing in the background while shadows from the screen danced on the walls. I didn't want to scare Kathy, so I stood across the room and softy called her name. She mumbled and rolled over, facing the opposite direction. I called her name louder and she turned over and looked at me with a strange look on her face.

I reached for the phone to call Maggie when Kathy yelled out not to touch it. Her tone gave me chill bumps.

"What on earth is wrong with you? What do you mean don't touch it? It's not a snake. It's a telephone."

"Just don't. Don't listen to the message, Jenny, please," Kathy pleaded.

"Look, no matter who it is, if there's a message, I need to hear whatever they say, and you need to get up.

What the heck is she talking about a message when the light isn't blinking? We have to go to Maggie's office as soon as possible. We're going to have a meeting with both her and Steve. I hope we can work together to come up with a plan."

"But if you listen to the message, you won't want to stay for a meeting. Maybe you'll want to pack up and leave immediately."

Kathy hovered in front of the phone to block me so that I couldn't press the message button. I was annoyed. After my conversation with Maggie, I just wanted to get a plan in place so we could all move forward, but Kathy continued to antagonize me about this phone message.

"You act so paranoid at times. I don't think it's warranted 24/7. It begins to wear on one's nerves after so long."

I angrily moved her out of my way.

"Have it your way, Jenny. Play the flippin' message. Play it!" she exclaimed.

She had succeeded in making me extremely aggravated and antsy, but I needed to see what the hullaballoo was all about. I listened as the words cut into me like a sharp knife.

"Remember what I told you girls a long time ago? You can't run away from The Group; not now, not ever. You see, we are everywhere. Yes, you heard me… everywhere. Oh, and by the way, tell Maggie Claire and Steve Green that I am looking forward to seeing them, too." Click.

"Okay, what did I tell you?" Kathy asked. She darted around the room stuffing her clothes into her suitcase. "Did you think I was dramatizing something as serious as this? Well, now you know.

You heard for yourself. There's no way to escape and nowhere to go."

I didn't know how to respond to her or to anything. She was right. I wished I hadn't played the message.

"Communicate your brilliant ideas now, Jenny. What do we do?"

"There's nothing we can do," I replied sullenly. "We might as well quit. This thing is bigger than we know. We've reached the end."

"What do you mean quit? Give up to The Group that's killing, implanting chips and doing sinister things to so many innocent people? Quit, you say? How can you talk like that? You, who preaches that people should fight the impossible fight? What's gotten into you?" Kathy shouted.

I stared off into space. I was ready to throw in the towel.

"Maybe we should go back to Morganville and take our old jobs back. I don't know how to fight them. How can we fight? We don't even know what we're fighting. Don't you see where I'm coming from?" I asked without looking at her.

"No, Jenny. I don't."

I knelt down so I could be face-to-face with her.

"Kathy, I'm mentally whipped. Never would anyone have convinced me in the past that those words would come from these lips, but this is a conspiracy group with co-conspirators that span the globe. They've managed to conceal themselves, which tells me we haven't a chance in hell. There's no need for us to discuss this issue any further. It's time to go meet Maggie and Steve."

"But, Jenny, I..."

"Kathy, let's go."

I stood up and put my hand out to help her up. The phone rang as we opened the door to leave. I looked at Kathy as she looked at the phone. I eased the door shut after we exited the room. We no longer cared about who was calling.

I knocked on the office door. The door opened without anyone saying a word. It was as if it had opened on its own. Maggie and Steve were sitting on the couch with horror-stricken looks on their faces. As Kathy and I stepped in, the door slammed behind us.

"Welcome, girls. It's my pleasure to see you both again. You left town without saying goodbye. This hurt us so deeply. How could you think so little of us to do this dreadful thing? I know you must feel some repentance regarding your actions."

Dr. Kenalog eased toward us as we grabbed for each other's hand and walked backwards into the room.

He continued, "We have a motto in The Group: Forgive and Go Get. We've had this little issue before, you see. Take a seat with the good psychiatrist and her know-all brother. I need to establish a few things so we can move on."

"How dare you!"

Steve jumped out of his seat defensively, but one of Dr. Kenalog's henchmen responded quickly pushing him back down into his place.

"Sit down, Steve. Don't make me have to offer you a little help from my friends."

Shock swept over me. Kathy and I took a seat next to Maggie and Steve. From the looks on their faces, I felt reassured, more than ever, that they weren't in on this conspiracy.

Dr. Kenalog sat facing the four of us. Those cold, black eyes radiated a flicker of satisfaction that sent chills through me. Two men stood still and rigid, like toy soldiers, on either side of the doctor. A dark luminescence radiated from the men. Suddenly, I felt like laughing hysterically. The feeling rose up from deep in my gut. I fought to keep it at bay. I knew I had to maintain a modicum of control. I took deep breaths as Dr. Kenalog began to speak.

"Steve, Maggie, and, of course, Jenny and Kathy, let this little meeting come to order. This will be brief. You'll be taken to the airport this evening at 7:30 sharp. A private plane will transport you to the outskirts of Switzerland, to an island called Isle di Brissago. When you reach your destination, someone will take you to your quarters.

There are no phones in the rooms. Your meals will be served in a common room.

"Once in the common room, you will notice a monitor in the upper-left corner. This is a closed-circuit television. You will observe a screen coming down from the ceiling. Please take careful note of the docudrama. When it's over, someone will come to escort you to an underground level of the compound several floors below your sleeping quarters. You will ask no questions. The docudrama is crucial to your understanding what is expected of you."

Dr. Kenalog's cell phone interrupted him. The four of us sat as still as statues. He didn't stop staring at us during his brief conversation with God only knows who. This man had an overwhelming power over us and he took full advantage of it. He finished his call and stood up.

"On that note, I will leave you. The agenda that I have laid out for you will take place in precise order of time and travel, and will be adhered to with promptness. Problem conduct will not be tolerated by anyone. My advice to all of you is simple: Don't instigate problems or you'll get more than you can handle. Cooperate and the future could prove to be pleasant. You all have been chosen for a specific job because of your various abilities; so heed my warnings."

He turned and walked out as if nothing mattered. He was followed closely by his soldiers, who looked as though they had just walked off the set of a science fiction movie. We were all too stunned to speak. Somewhere in the distance, a loud clap of thunder broke the silence along with our hypnotic trance.

CHAPTER TWENTY-FOUR

The sky was painted a cerulean color. A lazy parade of white billowy clouds floated past my window. The early morning sun smiled down as if a weighty secret had been hidden inside Mother Nature's magic box. I listened for sounds coming from downstairs that would signal Mom and Dad were up, but it was unusually quiet. It was one of my favorite times of the year. Easter meant candy, pretty-colored eggs, and bunnies. Mom would hide fancy trinkets inside each plastic egg. As I became older, the gifts became appropriate for my age. Mom continued to make baskets. There were always tasty things to eat, and beautiful things to wear. Dad would sneak chocolate candies and eat them when Mom wasn't looking. She always had him on a diet, or so he let her think. Earlier in the week, she and Dad were whispering about where to hide my Easter gift. They said it was too large to hide.

I would be moving to another town in the next couple of weeks. This would be my last Easter at home with my parents before starting a new job and career. It was the last time I could pretend to be a little girl.

On Easter, we'd always gone to sunrise services. It would be dark when we'd leave home. The air would be cool and crisp. We would sing Easter hymns as the sun made its way across the rippling water. Dad would say a word or two. I always felt little goose bumps all over me when we started to pray.

Mama always said, "Jenny, I always tell you it will be cold down by the water, but you always forget your jacket."

I would smile because I never forgot my jacket. I just wanted to show off my new Easter dress. Dad would wink because he knew me inside out. I had never fooled him for one second.

"Jenny, would you come down, dear? It's time to eat, sweetheart. I have prepared some of your favorites."

"Okay, Mom, I'm on my way."

I ran down the stairs. Daddy had the front door opened wide. Outside, I saw a new convertible with ribbons tied around it. It was candy apple red.

Mom and Daddy came up behind me, put their arms around my waist, and said, "Happy Easter, Jenny. We love you, honey."

"Jenny. Jenny, what's wrong with you? Can you hear me? Answer me, do you hear me?"

I jumped up from the chair startled and in a daze. I had forgotten for a precious moment where I was and what was happening. I had taken a mental journey to my childhood and didn't want to come back to the place where evil things lurked in every other person we met.

We sat in Maggie's office, not saying a thing. Kathy was trying to talk to me. Her face reminded me of a clown with an evil grimace.

Nothing mattered to me. The cards had been dealt to us. Dr. Kenalog had found us.

"Jenny, what are we going to do? Talk to me. You've always had answers to every quandary we've been involved in," Kathy said.

"There are no answers Kathy. Can't you see that it's over for us? Please, be quiet. It wouldn't hurt if you prayed. If there's a God of this universe, call upon him now."

I stared out the window secretly wishing I could re-enter my Easter daydream.

"Maggie, do you or Steve, have any answers?" Kathy asked.

Steve replied, "Kathy, I hate to put it in this manner, but I must say this to all of you here. I personally feel this is a conspiracy that surpasses any of our intellectual abilities to comprehend. All of you need to understand that this isn't an occasional case of a small-scale group of people, in a few states, selling organs for quick money. We're fully aware that microscopic implants are playing a crucial role in what's taking place. Each one of us in this room has been involved in some way. Jenny, you and Kathy were in the hospital assisting with the organ program. You've seen things that you have not talked with Maggie or me about, but you have been involved and are involved deeper than you know. This thing was cleverly put together by a mastermind somewhere.

"As a lawyer, for some of the accident patients I have represented, I have taken the initiative, on numerous occasions, to do undercover work in and around the arenas of scientific experiments. In conferring with fellow professionals, we've reached a conclusion that we're dealing with mind-control organizations. Are we aware of who is involved in this sort of thing or why they're doing it? No, it could be a toss-up between military oppositions or maybe someone who holds a powerful position in our country; or possibly someone who we think of as our ally. I can tell you this for certain: It isn't beneficial to any of us, but it is obviously of considerable benefit to a group of unknown origin.

"In the early 1800s, Sweden, along with other countries, hid vital documents involving mind control and torture. They did things to patients without their permission. Today, cybernetic studies far surpass early experiments of bygone times. I'm apprehensive about what's to take place tonight and about our future."

Kathy sat on the couch hanging on Steve's every word. I continued looking out the window. I was so sick and tired of all this and I just wanted to go back in time. I wished I would've never taken Kathy up on her dare to meet those men in the diner. That meeting seemed like it happened a lifetime ago. Steve continued without taking a breath.

"I recall an astute, intellectual colleague of mine, Bear Sutton, speaking at a seminar a few years back. His message left an indelible impression on me, and I believe it's for all of us sitting here nursing our individual fears.

He said, 'A person of fear dies many times, but a brave person dies but once.' Choose your death, ladies, with those words in mind. We are now three hours away from our appointed destination. Individually, we must make peace with God, just as we must choose how many times we will die."

I had had enough of his not-so-uplifting talk. I turned and eyed Kathy hoping she would be able to read my agitated thoughts. I was relieved when she ended her one-sided conversation with Steve to switch her focus onto me.

"Jenny, let's go to our room. I don't know what else to do or say. We'll talk, or we won't talk. C'mon," Kathy said.

"Wait a minute." Maggie stopped us. "If you and Kathy go to your room, then how are we going to plan an escape before they get here to pick us up? Don't you think we should try to do something about getting out of here?"

"Maggie, didn't you hear what your brother said? All of his findings indicate that we are trapped. We have no way out. No, we can't see them, but somehow they can see us. Face it, whatever they are going to do to us or with us, will happen. We're finished," I replied.

"But, maybe not. Maybe there's some way out of this. Steve, tell her there's hope for us," Maggie begged.

Steve walked over to his sister and hugged her. He spoke softly as he took a relaxed position on the couch.

"Maggie, let them go to their room and be alone. They need to organize their feelings just as you and I do. You're grasping at straws. Let's sit and talk for a little while. You must try to be strong."

He motioned to her to sit next to him. Maggie was angered by all of our responses. She wasn't about to surrender to the bullies.

"All right, Steve, damn it! Give up, then. Sit here and tell me about some farfetched plan of the government or some genius somewhere typing in radio frequency IDs."

"Maggie, this is not about RFID tracking. It's far more advanced than that."

Kathy was fueled by Maggie's fire. She agreed wholeheartedly that we shouldn't give in, but still we needed time to regroup.

"Let's go, Jenny. I'm like Maggie; I want to fight, but how?"

We walked out of the office but not before seeing tears streaming down Maggie's face. Steve was trying to comfort her, but his face gave way to his own true feelings. We all had to face death. Fear was overwhelming us and winning the battle. I unlocked the door to our room and entered. The light on the phone was blinking. I had no intention of checking it, and I felt sure Kathy wouldn't either. I turned on the lamp and sat down. Kathy sat down on the chair across from me.

"Jenny, you know we could always just take our own lives before they do. This sounds crazy, but it will at least keep us from torture or whatever they are going to do to us later."

I was shocked that she'd suggest such a thing.

"Kathy, you're a nurse. How can you talk like that? I would have never thought that you would be the type of person to entertain thoughts of suicide. No, I will do no such thing and neither will you."

I repeatedly glanced at the clock on the wall which was ticking louder than usual. The sun had gone down leaving behind a blanket of grey mist. It was getting close to the time.

"Do we finish packing, or do we just walk out of here? What do we do?" Kathy asked.

"I don't know. We take nothing; I guess."

"Jenny, we've got at least an hour and a half before they arrive. Why can't we leave and go somewhere in the mountains? We could change our looks so they couldn't recognize us. We could join a convent in one of those secluded areas and become nuns. That would be perfect for us."

Kathy became excited over her latest attack of brilliance.

"So what do you think we should tell Maggie and Steve? Are you suggesting we just vanish and say nothing to them?"

"Yes, Jenny, it's not like we're close friends. We haven't even known them for a week. Yes, I think we should leave, but we would have to figure out how to get away without them knowing."

I thought about her idea for a moment. I was never a spontaneous person, but I also never faced this level of danger before. We really had nothing to lose at this point. As far as we were concerned, our lives were over anyway. This could be our only chance to get away.

"If they spot us leaving, we could just tell them that we want to take a last minute ride before everything goes down tonight. Once we get away from the inn, we head to Vegas and catch a flight to somewhere far from here."

I nodded in agreement. I was relieved my car wasn't damaged from the flood like I thought it would be. Once it was dried out and cleaned, they brought it to the inn and parked it in the garage for us. My last Easter present would be our lifesaver. We had to at least try to escape.

"All right, let's go," I replied. I snatched my car keys off the dresser. "Just grab your purse. That's all we're taking."

We stepped out into the hallway just as another guest came out of his room. He nodded before heading down the hall toward the main entrance. We walked toward the dining area as he turned into the hallway leading to the registration desk.

"We'll go through the dining room and out the side exit. It's dinnertime so the place should be bustling. We won't even be noticed. Maggie and Steve are probably still talking in the office. We should have a clear shot to the exit."

"Look, Jenny, there's Steve on the phone, but his back is turned. Hurry before he turns around."

We hurried out the side door without drawing any attention to ourselves. There was a chill in the air as lightening sailed across the dark sky in front of us. The car was in the parking garage. It was only a short distance from the main building.

"Jenny, wait!" Kathy stopped me. "See that man walking over there by the corner?" She pointed up to the top of the parking garage.

"Yes, I see him now. Oh no, it's not a man Kathy. Look, it's Maggie! Why would she be out here?"

"This is too bizarre, Jenny. Well, we don't have time to follow her. We've got to go. She's out of sight anyway. Hurry, so we can get to the airport quickly. We're wasting time."

We edged along in the shadows until we reached the stairwell. Neither of us was wild about climbing the stairs in the dark. We were half way up the first level when we heard muffled sounds in the distance.

"Did you hear that?" Kathy asked.

"Yes, I heard it. I couldn't quite make it out, but maybe it was a car backfiring somewhere on the main road. Let's hurry. Get up the steps. I don't like it in here."

I tried to get her to move faster, but instead she turned to head down the stairs. Kathy started to panic.

"We better go back and forget this. Let's just go back," she said.

I grabbed her arm to stop her on the second-floor landing.

"No, Kathy, there's no turning back now. We don't have that far to go, anyway. Look, we're almost to the third level. Let's hurry. This place gives me the creeps."

With hearts pounding, we made it to the third floor. I knew the car was on the top level against the far wall in row D. It was a few feet away in a darkened corner. I felt a pang of dread go through me, but I knew we had to get to my car. We were in row C when I saw it. There was a light on inside my car that looked like a reading light. It was by the rear door on the passenger's side.

"Oh, no, Jenny, there's Maggie sitting in the back seat of your car. What do we do? She's obviously on to us."

Kathy was freaking out. There was no time to waste. I was determined to leave with or without Kathy, and Maggie, if necessary.

"Fine, if that's the case we'll just tell her our plans. I don't care. Maybe she'll go. Have you considered that maybe that's what she's here for? She's on our side. We'll talk to her, and she can decide if she wants to come with us. If not, then she can get out of the car. It doesn't matter to me."

I was hoping to settle this with Maggie as quickly as possible.

"All right, you talk to her, Jenny. I'll get in on the other side."

It wasn't until we reached the front doors of the car that we noticed the splattered stain that tainted the vehicle's interior. Kathy and I saw Maggie's lifeless body at the same time. There was a hole in her forehead. Blood spilled down her face and pooled onto her folded hands. A note had been placed between her fingers. It was written in bloody words that would never be read. Her blank eyes stared straight ahead.

CHAPTER TWENTY-FIVE

Why had we been foolish enough to think we could get away? I couldn't get Maggie's face out of my mind. *Why was she in my car?* There was something ludicrous about the thought, but we would never know. They had warned us not to cause any problems, but what had she done to deserve this? We didn't have time to stand here hashing out the whys.

"Kathy, let's get back to the office to see Steve before we have to leave for the airport at 7:30."

When we got back to the office, we found Steve in total shock. He already knew. None of us were able to utter a word about Maggie. I wanted so much to talk to him, but I felt too sick. We left her just as we had found her. Both of us were hysterical. A phone call had alerted him of things he wouldn't reveal. He didn't move a muscle. Anyone with a shred of understanding could tell he was weighed down with agony. His words would forever be locked up behind eyes full of pain.

I thought of Frank, Maggie's fiancé, and wondered if he had any idea about her involvement in this mess. Regardless of whatever he knew or didn't know, he would be devastated when he found out what had happened. I wondered when they would find her body in my car. *Does that make me a murder suspect on top of everything else?* Not that it mattered, but I hoped that Frank knew in his heart that we had nothing to do with the crime.

He saved our lives and we unknowingly led murderers right to Maggie's doorstep. What a cruel turn of events!

It was 7:30 sharp. The office door opened. The men resembling toy soldiers entered. There were four of them. They stood all around us. We were ushered out the door in single file. Not a word was uttered. We walked a few feet before reaching the car. I hoped Kathy would refrain from any outbursts. She had pulled herself together for the past few weeks and appeared to be mentally prepared for the worst. I hoped I could do the same.

Someone nudged me to get in the car. I slid across the seat and reached out in the darkness to the hand that touched mine. It was Kathy. She had always worn her watch with the face on the inside of her wrist. It was a nurse thing. She grabbed my hand but said nothing. Steve moved in to my left. He took my hand and squeezed it firmly as well. It was so dark in there. The windows were heavily tinted. It was dark outside too. The moon was not out and the desert was void of any lights. I couldn't see my own hand in front of my face.

As the car moved, we couldn't see or hear the men because a dark window stretched across between the front seat and the back seat. Our view was also blocked by a curtain. I felt as if someone had taken me into a time warp. Maybe this would all be over soon. Maybe I was in hell.

We seemed to have traveled for miles. I sensed at least an hour had passed when we came to an abrupt halt. None of us said a word. Without further explanation, we were told to get out of the car and we walked in single file. We boarded a plane. A harsh voice instructed us to take a seat. I sat down wondering what to expect next, when something came around my waist. I sucked in my breath as the metal belt made a clicking sound. A female voice assured me that it was only an electrically charged seat strap and that it was harmless, unless we decided to cause the crew problems while in flight. I could hear Kathy directly behind me. The female voice was telling her the same thing about the seat belt. Kathy barely talked in a whisper as she tried to respond. The roar of the engines was deafening. At any other time, it would have been a pleasant sound, but tonight it sounded like a demon's howl. I could not explain the feeling that churned in the pit of my stomach. I wondered where they had taken Steve. At least I knew where Kathy was.

A voice came over the loud speaker. It was another female.

"Ladies and gentlemen, your electronically charged seatbelts are secure for takeoff. You will be allowed to move about the plane after we turn off the seatbelt sign; however, you will not be able to get up until I release your belts from my control panel. I have full control of you from here on. You have no reason to be afraid as long as you fully understand the significance of the word "cooperate." It is in your best interest not to force me to use other methods.

Those seatbelts are an ingenious invention, and I can assure you, I don't mind using them. Let's make this the easiest flight possible."

Once we were in the air, a few people took positions in each of the aisles. I looked at the face of the man who stood directly above me. I knew his face, but I could not place it at the moment. He was one of the toy soldiers who'd taken us from the inn. His face, however, was all too familiar. It made me feel even more uneasy than I already was.

Eventually the stress of all that had happened caught up with me and I fell into a deep and dreamless sleep. When I woke up I figured we had to be close to our destination. We could've easily been flying for several hours.

"Jenny, are you in front of me? I can't see over the seats," Kathy whispered.

"Yes, Kathy, it's me. Try to stay calm."

"I'm doing my best," she replied.

"May we talk to each other now?" I asked the toy soldier who stood over me in the aisle.

He smiled his porcelain grin at me.

"Yes, Jenny, of course you may. I will alert the captain that all is well, and you may get up and move about the cabin."

"How did you know my name? Do I know you?

Have I worked with you at one of the hospitals?" I was still struggling to put all the puzzle pieces together.

"Yes, oh, yes, little Jenny girl. You know me, but not from the hospital; no, not from the medical world at all. It'll come to you in time. You'll figure it all out soon."

With that remark, he turned and walked away. I realized my seat belt had been released and I was free to stand. I looked around. I had never seen an airplane of this size. It looked like a huge room in a house. There were curtains on all of the windows in a variety of strange colors. There was an adjacent room winding around on the other side. The door was closed and there was a sign on it written in large red letters that said 'Do Not Enter.'

I stood in the aisle to talk to Kathy who remained in her seat.

"Kathy, did that man call your name?"

"No. Did he call your name?" she asked.

"Yes, he said he knew me and that I knew him. I know that I do, but I can't figure from where. He said I would know soon enough. How odd. It's just another dark spot in this thing."

"Jenny, Kathy, may I join you?" Steve asked as he walked up behind me.

I turned and clasped my hands around his hand.

"Oh, Steve, we're so sorry for what happened to Maggie. I know there's nothing we can do but offer our condolences."

He nodded graciously and looked down with sorrow.

"There's nothing any of us can do now but face what lies ahead." He looked back and forth at each of us and said, "I just want you both to know that you are wonderful ladies and it's been an honor to know you. I have grown fond of you both in this brief period of time.

"Kathy, I apologize that you and I started out on the wrong foot. You still remind me so much of my wife. I miss her, and guess I always will."

"Steve, it's forgotten, my friend. All is well as far as I am concerned. I wish things weren't as they are now."

"Steve, you look so weary. Is there anything we can do for you?" I asked.

"No, no, Jenny. There's nothing anyone can ever do again, I'm afraid."

The door opened to the other side of the cabin, and a faint glow emanated from the room. The shadow from it danced on the ceiling. I could hear music, but nothing I had ever heard before. It was almost angelic. A figure from inside the room stood in the doorway and motioned to one of the tin soldiers. The figure had on a long robe that covered it from the neck down to the floor. The soldier walked into the room and closed the door behind him. A female appeared from the cockpit and walked up and down the aisle. She said nothing to us and we didn't say anything to her.

"Jenny, did you see that robed person who stood in the doorway? And that music; how strange was that music? It was as if angels were playing it, but there are no such things on this earth."

"Oh, for sure, Kathy, I saw it, all right. They certainly wanted to guard their identity for some reason."

"Steve, do you have more insight into this group than you've been telling us?"

"I'd rather not say, Jenny. I have my ideas, but I don't have enough conclusive evidence put together to discuss any of it. It doesn't matter. I know there's nothing we can do. I haven't been able to comprehend the magnitude of this thing. Quite honestly, it overwhelms me."

Our discussion was interrupted by one of the soldiers.

"Ladies and gentlemen, take your assigned seats. The seat restraints will automatically lock within a few seconds after you are situated. We will begin our descent in a few minutes. You will remain seated until I unlock your seatbelts."

After a brief good-bye, Steve and I returned to our seats. I assumed it wouldn't be long before we'd finally face the rulers of this whole nightmare and possibly greet our demise.

CHAPTER TWENTY-SIX

I fell into dark brooding. None of this made sense to me. We were held captive with electrically charged seat belts. If any of us made the wrong move, we would be given a jolt of electricity like that of an electric chair. I was not sure if it would kill us or serve as just a warning. I could hear Kathy behind me. She was whispering or praying, which we all needed to do. Steve was directly behind her.

It seemed like only yesterday when Kathy and I were laughing at each other. We had decided to go skiing in Colorado. Neither of us had ever been on a pair of skis. We were both clumsy, but skiing proved to be an accomplishment after all because we didn't kill ourselves the first day. She was quick to remind me of the time we had signed up for parachute jumping. She landed on her leg and twisted her ankle, which left her with a fracture. Those memories were part of us. Tears welled up in my eyes and spilled down my cheeks. *At least they couldn't take our minds or the memories stored safely inside, or could they?* For now, we could take our memories from their chambers and gaze upon them at random.

The pilot's voice came over the loud speaker.

"We'll be landing in five minutes. You'll stay seated until someone escorts you from the plane. Do as you are told, and there'll be no problems. Do not force us to vary from protocol. We do not tolerate disobedience."

The plane made its descent and jolted on landing. I sat quietly, digging my fingers into the arms of my seat, wishing for a quick and painless end to this scenario. With my heart pounding like a hammer, I felt the seat belt release. My breath seemed to be trapped in my lungs. *Where were the people in the other room, and who were they? Better yet, what were they?* I felt a hand on my arm. A female voice spoke quietly but sternly.

"Stand up, Jenny. We have reached our destination. I will be directing you across the grounds to the place where you will be staying. You will be there for an undesignated amount of time."

I heard a male voice behind me talking to Kathy. She made no attempt to respond. I was worried about her. She didn't have the capability to deal with this kind of stress. Nursing stressors were one thing, but this was a whole different world. I heard Steve talking in the background. His voice was chillingly calm. I wondered if it was because he was a man or a lawyer who had faced unexpected challenges many times. Maybe he had resigned himself to accept the inevitable. In the courtroom, lawyers play one role in trying to convince the jury. They play another role in counseling their clients. They have to rise to the occasion, and I guess that's what Steve was doing.

"Okay, take the steps as quickly as you can. We have a schedule to keep. Kathy, you'll descend the steps behind Jenny, so be sure to move quickly."

With that, Kathy got to her breaking point.

"I can't do this. I am not moving. Do you hear me? This is the most absurd thing in the world. I'm not taking another step until you explain where you're taking us and why. We have rights just like all of you do. Now, what are you going to do, shoot me perhaps? Microchip me right here on the steps? Yeah, that's a brilliant idea. Do it now."

"Follow my orders, Kathy, or you will regret it," the female guard said.

"Miss Guard, may I please talk with her?" I asked. "Please?" I begged. "I will do exactly as you say, but give me one moment with her. Just one moment…" I didn't wait for the guard's approval; instead I pulled Kathy aside by the arm. "She's just upset that's all. She'll be fine after I talk to her."

I nodded my head in assurance, hoping the guard would copy the motion.

"All right, make it quick, or I can handle it quite well my own way," the guard replied.

I pulled Kathy further aside and whispered directly into her ear.

"Kathy, look it's going to be okay. Listen, we will be in the room in a short time and we'll be together. C'mon now, take a deep breath, and do what they want. It's all going to change shortly. Okay?"

She pulled back from me.

"But why are they doing this, Jenny? Why?"

I stared directly into her eyes and spoke as calmly as I could.

"I don't know the answer to that question. I do know it's better to follow their orders. You don't want things to be harder than they already are. Just act as if you're following protocol at the hospital. You know there were times when we didn't always agree with the docs, but we did what we were told. Right? Just do it for now."

"Okay, Jenny, fine.... I won't say anything else; at least not right now."

The guard who was escorting me was annoyed. She pulled me back into line.

"All right, Jenny. You did your good deed for the day, now move along. They're waiting on us. You've wasted enough time coddling her."

I didn't break eye contact with Kathy until the last possible second. We walked down the steps of the plane and took a right as directed. We walked a couple of blocks with the tin soldiers by our sides. They weren't actually made of tin, but they walked stiff and robotic, spoke with a broken speech like something animated, yet they were humans, I thought. I could hear Steve mumbling in the background. The voice talking to him sounded familiar, but I couldn't put a face or name with it. I didn't want to, really. The lead guard stopped the line from moving once we reached a large gate.

"We are now at the institute. We will proceed to the elevator that will take us to your quarters where you will remain until further notice. You've been briefed already on the docudrama."

"Will we be sharing the same room?" I asked.

"Yes, as a matter of fact, you will. As I said, you'll be watching a brief docudrama. It includes images of what we're about to show the world. You won't understand what you're seeing, but it's a beginning."

The guard entered a code into a control panel, sending a buzzer into a loud frenzy. I jumped and stifled a scream. I was nudged to step forward through the gate. It was a short distance to the elevator. I stepped inside and walked to the back as directed.

"Kathy, hang on, okay? Here, take my hand. Just know that we'll be together. Together we can do whatever needs to be done. You know the old saying about a house divided will fall. Just stay with me."

"I will. I'm sure we'll find out that it's actually not as bad as we have made it."

Kathy squeezed my hand.

"Steve, are you with us?" I asked.

"Yes, Jenny, I am. You girls try to hang tight. It's true what they say about houses divided, so if we stick together, we'll make it.

We must keep level heads." Steve called out from the front of the elevator.

We were packed in like cattle. It seemed like we rode up several floors before the elevator finally stopped.

"We've reached our destination; step out and turn left," said the lead guard.

We walked in single file. The tin soldiers surrounded us all the way. The sound of keys rattling announced that we had arrived at our quarters. The door opened. An unusual music wafted in the air—it reminded me of the music on the plane. The sounds were impossible to describe and I don't know that they've ever been heard on this planet. I felt as though a vacuum was pulling me into its clutches. Words formed, but my lips wouldn't move as I tried to speak. We looked around the room. The furnishings were like the music in that descriptions would be impossible. The colors of each piece of furniture were astonishing. The room seemed to hold its own magnetic lure as it silently drew us into another place and time. I felt hypnotized; however, I knew I had to maintain some semblance of alertness and sanity.

The guards who brought us here had already left the room, shut the door, and locked it. A door opened in the back of the room. A figure in white entered then stood in the center of the room. It was as though a spirit of another world had filled the space with an awesome presence. There was peace and calmness around the figure.

"Your dinner will be served soon. Won't you please take a seat?"

We all sat down simultaneously without saying a word. We were mesmerized by the décor, music, and the angelic figure in white, her voice as soothing the colors. The music continued to seek out our minds, as if to release us from all thought processes. We were rendered helpless, both mentally and physically. The figure in white disappeared through a door with the number six painted on it. The color of the number spoke its own language. Everything around us had numbers, letters, or biblical symbols.

Suddenly, in the center of the room, the floor opened up like a trap door. A table came up from the opening. A voice drifted in with the music.

"Dinner is served."

Another door opened behind us. We turned around to see figures robed in gold carrying platters of food. The dishes were placed on the table in front of us. Not a word was spoken as they turned and quickly left the same way they had entered. The lights were dimmed, and a monitor appeared from behind a sliding door in the upper corner of the room.

I looked at Kathy and Steve. They were drinking something exotic. It was red in color and mixed with miniature blue and pink balls resembling marshmallows.

They had already started eating. Throughout our travels, the thought of food never crossed my mind. I couldn't even remember our last meal. The smell that wafted through the air was intoxicating. All of a sudden I was hungry and parched, but something about this set-up didn't seem right. Our captors couldn't be trusted.

"What are you eating and drinking?" I asked.

Kathy and Steve stuffed their faces and looked to be enjoying every bit of their feast. They didn't answer me.

"We have no way of identifying any of this. What makes you think it's safe?"

"Jenny, I can't speak for Steve, but we are here. I no longer care what any of it may or may not do. I will no longer dwell on anything as trivial as food or drink. And, to be honest, it is the most delicious food that I have ever placed in my mouth."

Steve nodded in agreement with Kathy since his mouth was too full to speak. I picked up a glass and filled it with the pink liquid from the crystal pitcher. Kathy was right. At this stage, how could eating exotic foods and drinks make anything worse than it already was? Just as I picked up my fork, the screen lit up and brightened the room.

A black background with flashes of red surged across the screen. There appeared to be ancient symbols, medieval codes, or something of that nature. We ate in silence, while staring at the screen. Figures donning masks were hooking wires to something that wasn't within view. To the right was another group of masked figures standing in front of a large wall that displayed an outline of the United States. Each state was pegged with symbols that resembled crosses, bibles, and other religious pieces. Every figure was intently working on the board while communicating in sign language.

Supposedly, we would understand our roles in The Group after viewing the docudrama. The light in the room, along with the music, seemed to be taking pieces of our minds, little by little. The mythological nectar of the gods had been fed to us. A screen that held the key to our life or death made no sense to any of us. Hooded figures without faces labeled the states with biblical icons. They were invading our brains and plugging them with odd symbols. The screen dimmed as the black background lit up with numbers that danced across in a fiery swirl. We were spellbound.

"Ladies and gentleman, you've just watched a brief excerpt of a world-wide phenomenon. There are specific reasons for your part in this. You will meet your superiors in the underground level. They will help you to better understand your role in this mission."

The screen disappeared in the same manner in which it was presented. The music stopped. White-robed figures came in to remove the food. All of a sudden, reality gripped me. We had been in a hypnotic state.

Had we just seen a film of weird happenings and actions or had we not? Did we eat, or was it all a mirage of some kind? I could no longer separate reality from fantasy.

"Jenny, what just happened?"

"I'm as dumbfounded as you are, Kathy. My ability to reason has become impaired."

"Steve, do you know what has taken place tonight, or is it morning? I don't even know whether it's day or night."

"I don't know, Jenny. I think it's some sort of subliminal propaganda. They have interspersed messages within the music, possibly, and maybe the drink. I can only say to you that if God doesn't deliver us, we are doomed."

"Do you think we're going to die, Steve?" Kathy asked.

"Not necessarily, but death is not always the worst scenario in every case. This is one of those times."

The main door opened, and in walked several hooded figures. They had come to take us to the underground level. They motioned for us to follow them.

"Jenny, why don't they talk to us instead of motioning?"

"They probably just have microchips and aren't programmed to talk."

They held the door open as we marched out like robots. They walked beside us, one by one. We went in groups of three. We reached the elevator, where we waited in silence for the next trip. The elevator stopped, and the doors slowly opened.

"Oh my God, Jenny. Oh my God."

Steve gasped and I, too, felt the air leaving my lungs. The elevator was pure glass. Seats came up from the floors. The inside seats were made of padded leather. The color was orange, yellow, and red. Mesmeric music floated through the door as we were nudged inside. The door closed behind us. Belts came around us much like the ones on the plane. They fastened securely as we started down the elevator shaft. A voice came from a speaker that appeared to surround us from the floor to the ceiling.

"Steve, Jenny, and Kathy, welcome to operation headquarters. We have begun our descent to underground operations. You will see nothing for a short time as we move."

"Jenny, I'm going to faint. My head is swirling."

"Take a deep breath, Kathy. We need to maintain composure as best as we can," said Steve.

"How can you say that?" I asked.

"Jenny, if they wanted to harm us, they have had numerous chances to do so. Don't you realize that long before now, months and months ago, they could have killed us or placed the chips in us? They didn't for some reason. They are saving us for something else."

The music became louder as though someone, or something, had heard our discussions. Maybe it was an attempt to hypnotize us before we became hysterical. Outside the elevator, the walls were dark as far as we could see. We rode in silence. It must have been an underground man-made place. The music seemed to lay curled inside the cubicles of our minds. A beam of light appeared from below the elevator. We were getting close.

"Jenny, do you see the light? It's a yellow glow of some sort." Kathy was frantic.

"Yes, yes, I see it. We're almost at the end."

The light became brighter as we neared the bottom. It began to surround us from every side. We tried to shield our eyes. The closer we moved to the center, the more blinding it became. We were headed beyond the light down into what looked like a large black hole. Its shape was circular. It resembled an inner tube or doughnut. It was a mammoth ring-shaped object with lights and wires extending out in every direction. The elevator came to an abrupt halt. We were now in the center of it. The wires reached as far away as the eye could see with circular button-like objects blinking in infinite colors. The area surrounding this monstrosity had no beginning or end. *How could any human or group of humans build something of this magnitude?* I wondered.

"You will note on all sides that there are wires and buttons used to do the work that must be done here. You will be able to view a model of our baby when you get to the lower level. You will be there in a few seconds. Someone will take you to the next destination."

We were speechless. None of us could look at the others. We were unable to take our eyes off of this gigantic thing. *How long had it been operating? Who built and controlled it?* I had so many questions.

The elevator began the descent to the next destination. The lights were so bright that we couldn't see anything other than the glow. The elevator suddenly stopped. We found ourselves in a dark area. All we could see was what appeared to be a long hallway, lit with nothing but candles. There were rows and rows of candles on each side of the hall. The elevator door opened, and we were met by a group of six figures in black-hooded robes. They looked like monks. They gestured for us to walk ahead of them.

"Jenny, I wonder if…"

"There's nothing to say, Kathy. I can't talk to you. At this point, I can hardly breathe. The air is strange. I feel a spirit of oppressiveness surrounding me."

Steve interrupted, "Jenny, it benefits us all to maintain a strong front. We must not let them feel that we are weakening."

He was starting to annoy me.

"Steve, I understand, and I agree, but I can't breathe. Something in the air is smothering me."

"It's pure nerves," he said. "Just take a deep breath. They're indicating for us to stop at the door. You must gut it up. We're about to learn all about The Group. The end is here, and the new beginning is about to greet us. Prepare yourselves."

The figures stopped and stood on either side of the door. A deep female voice commanded us to enter. The door automatically opened. What met our eyes was beyond description. It was a place so immense in size that I could not see its ending.

"Oh, my God, what kind of place is this?" I asked.

"I don't know. It looks like an ancient cathedral," Steve replied.

It was dark, and there were only small windows around the areas we could see. Slits of a faint glow of light could barely be seen. The style resembled that of a basilica. Far in the distance stood an altar that extended from the floor to far above that which the human eye could see. It was gothic in design. An astronomical wooden clock was built in the nave. "Borologium Birabile" was engraved in bold letters into the middle of the time piece. Carved in wood below the letters were human faces. The face in the center was larger than the others. Jewels embellished every detail of that particular face. Underneath the face read the words "Noster Deus."

"Steve, what does that mean, Noster Deus?"

"It's Latin, Kathy. It means Our God."

The leaders, or whatever they called themselves, were watching, but allowed us time to take in our surroundings. The place was quiet and empty. The figures that led us in had suddenly disappeared.

On the far side of the giant auditorium, in a room to the left, the word crypt was boldly written in red on what looked to be a monumental sarcophagus.

"Steve, what is that? I think it looks like a stone coffin or something."

"I think you're right Jenny. It is a coffin. My God, it is."

There was so much to see. We had no clue what to expect, but just as we turned to take a step, a voice spoke. It came from every corner of the cathedral.

"You'll walk down the long hallway to your left. Do so at this time. At the end of the hall you will see a door on your left. When you reach the black and red door, you will enter only after knocking with the rapper one time."

"Kathy, are you holding on? We are all about to die I suspect, but you're too quiet."

"I am sick, Jenny. I'm so sick that I wish I was dead. I can't take this. I can't."

"Okay, Kathy. C'mon, honey." I put my arm around her shoulders and walked next to her. "C'mon now, things are going to work out. Okay?"

She whimpered. Steve put his arm around her shoulder on the other side.

"It's time to move. Now!" The tremendous voice echoed throughout the room.

"Okay, ladies, let's do what we're told. Whoever is in charge here won't be playing from the looks of this setup. We're in this together, as Maggie used to say when we were kids."

We walked toward the hallway as instructed. We moved together as though we were one body with three heads.

"Oh, Steve, the hallway looks dark. Everything is lit with candles just like the coming out meeting at the hospital. Jenny, remember how the hallway and meeting rooms were lit with candles?"

"Yes, how could I forget?"

"Steve, do you remember the coming out meeting that Maggie told you about?" Kathy asked.

"Yes, I remember what she told me. Let's go, we don't want to antagonize them."

Steve spoke calmly but with a sense of urgency. I was thinking what he was thinking—let's just keep moving and do as we're told. Two bronze doors led to the hallway that would take us to another part of this bizarre place. As we walked through the doors, it was as though we had been transposed into the coldest part of the world.

"It's so dark in here, even with all of the candles," I whispered. I could see my breath in the air.

"You're right, Jenny. It's like a dungeon," Kathy replied.

We were almost at the end of the hallway. It was like walking the length of a football field. We finally reached the door that we were to enter. It was indeed black and red with a huge rapper. Steve reached out to lift the knocker, but Kathy grabbed his hand to stop him.

"No, Steve, please. We can't do this. I can't..."

She was a mess. She was sobbing uncontrollably. Steve tried to console her.

"Kathy we must. I fear the consequences from this organization would be severe. We must cooperate with whatever we are told to do."

"I know, but I can't. Maybe you and Jenny can, but I can't. Let them do what they want to you two, but not me. I'm getting out of here now."

Steve grabbed Kathy and turned her toward him. She struggled against his grip.

"Do you remember what they did to Maggie? Well, do you? Now get it together. You're stronger than that, Kathy. I know you are. Nurses are trained in composure management, now compose yourself!"

Kathy stopped fighting him. She knew he was right. Steve handed her off to me and she practically collapsed into my arms. Steve reached for the rapper and tilted it up.
He paused briefly then let it fall against the door. The door opened.

"Enter, please."

Kathy was holding onto me for dear life. Though I was supposed to be consoling her, I needed consoling from her in return. Despite the fact that she wasn't the bravest person, I was so grateful that I didn't have to go through all of this alone.

We hesitantly walked into the room. It was even bigger than the one that held the clock and coffin. A large balcony sat several feet high in the air. It was adorned with gold curtains. A long table draped in white linen sat in the center of the room. Goblets were set in place exactly 6 inches apart. The table looked to be at least a hundred feet long. Every chair was in line, spaced the same distance apart; all of the chairs were the same distance from the table.

"You will seat yourselves in the three selle percée provided for you."

"I can't move. I am shaking so badly. Help me someone," Kathy begged.

"I've got you, Kathy. Jenny, take my hand. The chairs are only a few feet away. C'mon, we can do this." *Need damn binoculars just to see half way down the table!*

"What Steve?"

"Nothing, Jenny, nothing."

We walked to the chairs that sat back from the long table. The chairs looked like a king should sit in them. We sat down. The room was dimly lit with soft lights that penetrated every square inch of the walls.

Music, barely audible, began to play. A violin hummed with such sadness that it overwhelmed Kathy. She began to cry once again. Steve looked dumbfounded. I was mesmerized. Suddenly a platform appeared from an area several feet behind the table. It was the size of the room in length. The image of this monstrosity was chilling. Curtains shimmering with silver emblems covered the entire length of the platform. The emblems were distinctly Roman numerals. The platform abruptly stopped moving. I could hear Kathy and Steve suck in their collective breath. I wasn't sure that I was breathing. The curtain opened slowly, allowing us to see a set of crimson velvet chairs. The feet were brass and looked like claws. They were exquisite. The platform itself was beyond description. From the right side marched black-robed figures. From the left came figures dressed in red. There were many in number. They stood in front of the chairs with their heads bowed as if in prayer.

Another platform came down from the upper level as the music played louder. It stopped just in front of the platform of robed figures. The curtain opened. A light surrounded a figure in gold. He removed his hood and stood silently. The other robed figures removed their hoods in unison. They bowed to him before seating themselves. He nodded to them before turning to us. His face looked bronze in color. His eyes seemed to beam with radiance as did the halo that appeared to surround him. He had a way about him that captured each of us along with all of those in the room. I had heard of such a man when I was a child in church and down through the years. He was angelic looking, but pure evil, all in wrapped in one. They called him the anti-Christ. I wondered if this might be him. His voice was captivating.

"Ladies and gentlemen, you're about to meet the master of this operation, but first you will be introduced to the president of the organization. You'll receive a brief introduction to the organization before your training starts. You'll be training a minimum of two years."

He sat down. The glow that shadowed him was mesmerizing and found its way inside my spirit. Another man stepped forward.

"Good evening, I am Arch Bishop Reynaldo Diamond. I preside over all major cities and states within the United States of America. I have colleagues who work closely with me around the entire globe. Each of the gentlemen seated in front of you rules from the priesthood of every denomination in the world. Some are from the recently-established New Macrocosm Churches, an unknown term to you up to now.

It's a new method of worship that evolved a few years ago in the private sector. You'll learn their procedures, beliefs, and by-laws soon enough.

"All of our leaders are high-ranking men and women from the world's largest religious organizations. The world, as you know it, no longer exists; our new government is already established, but there is still quite a bit of work to be done. You are familiar with microchips and the implantation of such. Now you are going to meet the Master."

From the rear of the room, the wall parted in the middle, unfolding outward like gargantuan doors. The lights were blinding. Wires running in every direction were connected to the source. Complex pieces of metal and gadgetry sat in front of us taking up miles and miles of space. *This was the Master? Is it an alien?* I was so confused. Even though the Arch Bishop was finally giving us answers, I now had more questions than ever.

"You will note the wires running to assorted parts of the Master. Each infinitesimal wire controls the microchips that are embedded in people around the United States, Russia, and China. They are part of the New World Monastic Order. Each person is programmed to do what is required of them by the mere pushing of a switch. The states will be governed by a religious sphere of influence determined by that area's particular leader, of course.

"The leaders here this evening will determine the choice for each state's new rules and religious laws. The people who are already embedded with our chips will act as big brothers. If a particular state fails to comply with their monastic order, it will see numerous plagues, floods, fires, drought, and famines. You see, we have, and we will continue to wean out citizens by whatever means necessary."

But why? I kept asking over and over in my head. *Why did these people, or creatures, or whatever they were, need to have control over us?* I was too afraid to ask.

Arch Bishop Diamond continued, "I know that each of you is wondering why you are here and why you have not been imbedded with a microchip. Kathy and Jenny, we know your work has been exceptional in the medical field. Steve, your work as an attorney has been astounding. We know your backgrounds from childhood until the present time. All three of you will be assets to our world-wide endeavor. You will work wherever needed and will do as instructed. You're not the only three chosen to serve our mission in this manner. You will meet your equals soon enough. If any of you fail to comply, you will suffer the consequences.

"None of you will be implanted with a microchip. Instead, we have greater plans in mind. You've already met some of our microchipped humans, and well, let's just say, they're a little bit awkward. Therefore, we will be using your uniquely human abilities to bring others into our fold. If you disobey, you will be placed in your own world of plagues equal to the severity of your actions.

We've built fortresses on gated islands that will become your private place of penalization if you choose to go that route. Trust me, you don't want to disobey. Oh, no, no. You would wish for death, but you will not die.

If we choose? What choice do we have in this matter? I was screaming on the inside. For the first time in my life, death seemed to be a better option than to continue living.

Arch Bishop Diamond inhaled a deep breath. He was beaming with pride at all that his group of minions had accomplished. Just then, a rumble from the depths of the earth shook inside the cavernous room where we were seated. The three of us held onto the table out of fear that we would be jarred out of our seats. Meanwhile the robed men sitting around us weren't fazed at all by the movement. Yet the ground was literally quaking.

The miles of wires leading out of the creature that they called "Master" twisted like octopus tentacles. I shrieked as the finger-like lines curled and flipped. *Could it be that their Master was alive?* It all seemed so unreal. Arch Bishop Diamond shouted to us over the sound of its enormous twisting movement.

"Now, I am honored and most pleased to introduce to you, the greatest and most powerful being in the Universe, our Master, and your future electronic leader: "Encryption's Wrath."

**Follow Jenny and Kathy thru the sequel,
En*cryption's Wrath*.**